Pain is Fantastic

Dr. Troy H. Peters

Copyright © 2018 Troy H. Peters D.C.

All rights reserved. No part of this publication may be reproduced, distributed, or transmitted in any form or by any means, including photocopying, recording, or other electronic or mechanical methods, without the prior written permission of the publisher, except in the case of brief quotations embodied in reviews and certain other non-commercial uses permitted by copyright law.

ISBN-10: 1986091341
ISBN-13: 978-1986091343

DEDICATION

I would like to dedicate this book to those who are still looking for the answer to their health questions. I hope the words in these pages encourage you to take action, both massive action and tiny action, towards knowing your body and its massive potential.

NOW IT'S YOUR TURN

**Discover the EXACT 3-step blueprint you need to become
a bestselling author in 3 months.**

Self-Publishing School helped me, and now I want them to help
you with this FREE VIDEO SERIES!

Even if you're busy, bad at writing, or don't know where to start,
you CAN write a bestseller and build your best life.

With tools and experience across a variety niches and professions,
Self-Publishing School is the only resource you need to
take your book to the finish line!

DON'T WAIT

Watch this FREE VIDEO SERIES now, and
Say "YES" to becoming a bestseller by
clicking on the link below or by putting it into
your web browser:

https://peterswellness.com/selfpublishing.html

Table of Contents

Acknowledgements

Introduction   1
       Why was this book written and for whom was it written?
       A little about the author

Chapter 1 - Is pain fantastic and why should you care?   8
       Pain and Pleasure
       Disease
       Subluxations
       The Three Causes of Subluxation
       Preventative Maintenance and the Automobile Analogy
       Our Built in Warning System
       Symptoms Simplified
       Muscle Memory
       X-rays
       Symptoms and Preventative Maintenance
       Medication and Sugar
       Consistent Relationship with Your Body

Chapter 2 - Understanding why our bodies hurt.   21
       Baseline
       Health Pyramid
       Master Control System of the Body
       History and Examination

X-rays
Get Checked

Chapter 3 - How long do I have to suffer with these symptoms?   25

Chiropractic Care Forever......or not
Your Pain and the Visual Analog Scale (VAS)
Subjective Input from the Patient (OPQRST)
Objective Tests
Your X-rays
Activities of Daily Living
Time Frame for Healing

Chapter 4 - What is your health worth?   57

Health Insurance Costs
Health Care or Sick Care
Do More for Yourself and Pay Less

Chapter 5 - Isn't my problem just tight muscles?   62

Massage Therapy
Myofascial Release Therapy
Sprain versus Strain

Chapter 6 - What are the short cuts to getting better and are you willing to participate?   71

Certified Personal Trainers
Sleep
Water
Foam Roller
Stretching

Exercise
Proper Eating
Reading
Thinking Time
Home Traction
Consistency and Time Management

Chapter 7 - What is with all the expensive tests?   91
Physical Examination
X-rays
MRI/MRA/CT

Chapter 8 - What is the structural foundation of the human frame?   95
The Foot
Your Foundation
Foot and Pelvic Connection

Chapter 9 - In what position should I be sleeping?   99
Blood Supply to the Spinal Cord

Chapter 10 - What do you the reader want and how can I help you get what you truly desire?   101
Accountability
What is Your Purpose Statement?
What is Your Vision Statement?
What is Your Why?
Rid Yourself of Contradictions

ACKNOWLEDGEMENTS

I want to thank my amazing wife Karie and our daughters, Isabella, Ashley and Nicole for their never-ending support in my efforts to be the best husband, father and businessman I can be.

I want to thank my many mentors and teachers whose books, videos and courses are a constant source of inspiration for me.

I want to thank my past, present and future patients who allow me to help them in their journey to better health and happiness.

I would like to thank my editor, Nicholas. Without his input, this book would not be the same.

Introduction

Why was this book written, and for whom was it written and who am I, the author?

I am writing this book to help people who have been in chronic pain, and to help those who have or will have injuries. I want to help people understand the choices they can make which will nurture them back to true health, as opposed to just thinking they are fine because the pain is gone. We must make sure that our nervous systems are functioning at their very best in order to live to our fullest potential. My hope and intention is that you will enjoy what I have put together. I hope that we can grow in our knowledge of ourselves, and those around us, to live happier, more fulfilling lives. I believe the way to do this is by listening to our bodies, and knowing how to respond to the body's messages.

When I read a book, I always like to know a little about the author's qualifications, to help me better understand where the author is coming from. So, let me tell you about myself.

My name is Troy H. Peters D.C., Q.N. I am a chiropractor. I am certified in Quantum Neurology

Rehabilitation and Applied Kinesiolgy. In my personal life, I am also a step father of one son Anthony (age 28) and the father of three girls, Isabella (age 14), Ashley (age 12) and Nicole (age 12). Yes, Ashley and Nicole are twins. Let me begin with mentioning that if you want a challenge try having three children in diapers, being a recent college graduate with over $120,000 in student loan debt and moving to an area where you do not know anyone.

A few years ago, when I finished working with a patient, she asked me a strange question: "What inspired you to become a chiropractor?"

At first, I wondered why my story mattered to her. But then I did tell her my story, and she helped me to realize that for many patients, knowing their doctor's story and understanding the WHY behind their doctor's dedication can be a source of comfort. Since then, as a doctor, I've realized the value of telling my story. **After all, isn't comfort something a doctor should provide for their patients, while we guide them through what can at times be a painful healing process?**

So, what inspired me to become a chiropractor? It is not a pleasant story. I grew up on a small 200-acre dairy farm in Minnesota. As a child, my mom always had to take me to the doctor. I was always getting colds, and I missed a lot of school because of stomach aches and the flu. But my biggest problems were severe stomach and digestive issues.

Then one month, things got really bad. Imagine not being able to have a bowel movement for a week. Now, double that, and imagine the crippling pain of all that waste built up inside of you. (I warned you it wasn't a pleasant story.) Even after a 2:00 AM trip to the emergency room, I was still suffering from intense gastrointestinal pain that would not go away.

My dad, as a dairy farmer, did a lot of physical labor, so he made frequent visits to the chiropractor. Shortly after my emergency room trip, he decided to bring me to the chiropractor to see if it would help me too. The experience literally changed my life. It was not a miraculous one-time fix, but Dr. Paul Otto put me on a care plan to correct the subluxations in my spine. He gave me some nutritional advice and within a couple of weeks, I felt like a new person.

But my story with pain management, in my own life, doesn't end there.

I was lucky enough to serve my country in the United States Coast Guard. Seven years of active duty, and six years as a reservist. During this time, I did not continue going to the chiropractor, because chiropractors were not part of the military healthcare system back then. I was able to go to night school and earn my Associates of Liberal Arts degree. I was able to use my education, military training, and a good friend's connections to land a job with a communications software company in Northern California.

After two years of working in Accounts Payable for a medium-sized corporation, something terrible happened. One evening at sunset, I was riding my motorcycle with my now-wife, Karie, on the back. I pulled up to an intersection near my home, slowed for the turn to make sure no cars were coming, and rolled on the throttle to make my right turn. I never saw the thin layer of sand covering my portion of the road which had been spilled during earlier construction that day.

My beautiful custom painted CBR900RR hit the ground hard, with me and my future wife going along with it. Luckily, we were not hurt too badly. We were able to jump up, not get run over by oncoming traffic, and I was able to get us home without further incident. My motorcycle received most of the damage... or so I thought, until I awoke the next day.

Karie was feeling fine, but I felt like my head was going to explode. This was unusual, since I never got headaches. Karie recommended I see her dad's chiropractor, Dr. Ron Ohler, so I called and went later that same day. After the exam, X-rays and a much-needed adjustment, I went home and slept for 14 hours straight. I awoke the next day feeling like a human again, and thankfully, my head never did explode.

This incident made me look back and think about how much the chiropractic care I received as a child helped me with my intestinal issues, and here I was as a young adult being helped once again. When I was a child I had thought, it would be great to be a chiropractor but how would a small-town farm boy be able to accomplish that? Well, I wasn't a small-town farm boy anymore, so I decided to look into what it would take to become a doctor of chiropractic. I reached out to one of the fourteen chiropractic schools in the country at that time, Life Chiropractic College West. I found out that I would need another 6 years on top of my associates degree to get my doctorate in chiropractic.

After some soul searching, meditation, thinking, planning, and writing, I decided I was going to do whatever it would take to become a chiropractor.

It has been 13 years since I graduated with my degree in chiropractic and I love what I do. I started my practice in Northern California and after two years I moved my practice to Arizona. Being from Minnesota, Arizona was and is still very appealing to me. I work hard to serve my community with chiropractic care. I do my best to balance my time between work and home, because kids really do grow up so fast.

Here in the United States, what we have is not healthcare, but rather, some amazing "Crisis Care." Our medical doctors and surgeons are fantastic. But the problem is that everyone waits until they are *in* crisis before they decide to make some changes in their life, and if a patient is not willing to make some dietary and lifestyle changes, then the doctor has no choice but to put them on cholesterol lowering medications, blood pressure medications, insulin injections, and so on.

This is why I am a chiropractor. In this role, I have the ability to help patients with the *cause* of their problem, not just the symptoms. I do this by addressing the nervous system — the master control system of the body. As far as I'm concerned, it is the best job ever.

It is my hope and desire that, as you read through these pages, you will become more familiar with your body and its signals for help. No matter where we are in life, we can always be better, both physically and mentally.

This book was created as a way to answer some of my patients' most valuable questions. Questions which come up for coaches and athletes, weekend warriors, moms and dads, grandmas and grandpas, coworkers and friends. The questions I have chosen are the ones that come up time and time again for new patients and with people I meet out in the community. Let us always remember that health is each individual's responsibility. Others may help and guide us, but our everyday choices from the past have lead us to where we are today and our choices of today will lead us to where we will be tomorrow and in the future.

Chapter 1

IS PAIN FANTASTIC AND WHY SHOULD YOU CARE?

For over a decade, people have sought me out to assist them with many different ailments. Some of the most common concerns I see with my patients are: migraines, headaches (which is a different animal from migraines altogether), neck pain, shoulder pain, mid-back pain, low back pain, hip pain, knee pain, foot/ankle pain, elbow pain, and wrist/hand pain.

You have probably heard of the Freudian Psychoanalysis Pleasure Principle. This is the old adage that people are motivated by seeking pleasure, and avoiding pain. **Unfortunately, most seem to be more motivated by avoiding pain than by seeking pleasure.** Imagine living a life of working for more and more pleasure, instead of just doing enough to avoid pain.

Imagine it this way: picture an employee who shows up, but stays under the radar of the management team, only doing enough work to squeak by. Compare this to an employee who shows up early, is always willing to go the extra mile, stays late, and does not complain about it — because he or she has their eye on the big picture. They know why they do what they do, and they are striving for more pleasure out of life, because every day is an opportunity for them to better themselves, and to live the life they envision.

With all of that being said, we must also maintain all areas of our lives. Can you imagine working so hard, for so long, to get where you want to be and when you get there, everyone you care about no longer wants to be there with you, because you did not take the time and energy to show them how much they mattered?

When chasing your dreams, you must always involve those closest to you, so they know that the end goal *includes* them. Actions and words have a huge impact on relationships and all relationships need attention: husbands and wives, friends and coworkers, sons and daughters, all of these relationships need attention to flourish.

The same can be said about our relationship with our body. Do you know your body? Do you care for it so that you can function at your best or do you do just enough to avoid pain and discomfort?

Like with a bicycle, motorcycle, car, truck or computer, we need to do preventative maintenance for our physical, emotional, and chemical needs.

Now, I know that "preventative maintenance" does not sound sexy. But then again, Dis-ease isn't so sexy, either. For those who haven't seen the hyphenated form of the word *disease* before, let me explain. All diseases signify a lack of *ease*, or flow, within and throughout the body, and this has a negative effect on our nervous systems, which control everything within our bodies. This lack of ease distresses the balance and flow within the body and causes *Dis*-ease.

As a chiropractor, my job is to identify subluxations in the joints of the body which cause neurological inhibitions throughout the nervous system. Then, once I've identified them, I work to remove them. A subluxation is when a joint between two bones does not allow full movement of those two bones, because of some physiological reason. These reasons can be narrowed down to three forms for simplicity's sake: emotional causes, chemical causes and structural causes.

An *emotional cause* of a subluxation is just what it sounds like. Think of the things in life that people find stressful: work, relationship issues, raising children, unemployment, financial issues, divorce, death of someone close, you get the picture. Everyone knows that these types of issues cause emotional damage, but what many don't realize is that they also can wreak havoc on our bodies, and cause us not to perform at our best. This is because emotional problems cause our energy to be used elsewhere in the body, in order to deal with the emotional stressors. This can especially impact people who do not have a good way to cope with emotional stress.

Chemical causes of subluxations are things which have to do with the chemical makeup of our bodies at the cellular level. By that, I mean everything from the air we breathe, to the food we eat. Also, keep in mind that our skin is the largest organ of our body. Everything you touch comes in contact with this organ. We must be aware of what goes on our skin, because if the item or chemical compounds are able to be absorbed by the skin, then our bodies must deal with these chemicals at a cellular level. How does our body deal with these daily chemical invasions? Well, our circulatory system is filtered by our liver. Our liver filters our blood like the fuel filter in a car. Without clean fuel, a car will not run well, and without clean blood, *we* will not perform well. So, watch what you eat, know what is in the air that you breathe and be aware of what products you put on or allow to touch your skin because it all affects how we perform.

Structural causes of subluxations are things such as a slip and fall, a roller coaster ride, sports injuries, and automobile accidents like the fall I took off my motorcycle, as mentioned before. These structural injuries create areas in our bodies that do not perform the way they were designed to perform. Injuries can cause ligament and tendon sprains and strains, and damaged muscles.

When we think of the joints of the body, let's think about bones, ligaments, tendons, and muscles. Now, don't worry, I'm not about to give you a biochemistry book for the classroom. But on the other hand, if I do not go into enough depth for you, please look up any of the terms I use for further, deeper understanding.

A ligament is a very strong tissue that connects bone to bone within the body. A tendon attaches muscle to bone. There are about 210 bones in the human body. There are about 650 muscles in the human body. Of course, we could break this down into further detail, but for our purposes, focusing on 210 bones and 650 muscles in the human body will suffice.

Now before anyone gets bored with the seemingly mundane information above, let's review why we are covering this material: namely, why are you having these symptoms? Going back to the preventative maintenance analogy, we can simply drop our car or truck off at the shop and let the mechanic fix it, but we should have some general guidelines as to when and why to drop it off at the shop in the first place.

Sticking with the car metaphor, the manufacturers are getting better and better at helping us maintain our vehicles. Take some of the basics that most everyone is familiar with. When the gas gauge shows that the fuel level is getting low, swing into the gas station and add fuel. We should rotate our tires about every 5,000 miles. We should change our oil about every 5,000 - 8,000 miles. Do you remember when all we had was a simple red oil light that would come on if the oil pressure dropped too low? Now we have gauges, which show the pressure of the oil, *along* with an oil light (idiot light) which help us to keep a closer eye on it. This is like the blood in our arteries and veins, which allows us to live. In cars, the oil allows our vehicles to drive down the freeway at amazing speeds, all the while keeping us cool or warm, comfortable and safe. **So, what type of gauges and warning systems does our amazing body come with?**

Isn't it fantastic that our bodies have a way of letting us know something is wrong? Well, one major warning signal is pain. We have a built-in system which gives us signals along the way, and if we ignore these signals, the ending result can be more *intense* pain. With blunt trauma, this injury process sets off our warning system extremely fast, and the pain feels instantaneous. Our human bodies come with idiot lights too, just like the old oil lights on our car dashboards. Like automobiles, we also have gauges and warning signs of how our bodies are running.

There are many other warning systems. If we do not get enough sleep, we become tired. So, being tired can be a symptom of not getting enough sleep. Now, being tired can mean a plethora of other things, but for right now, let's keep this simple. Are you getting the proper amount of sleep? Most recommendations for sleep are between seven-to-nine hours of sleep per night. Now, there are exceptions, but for our purposes we are going to go with seven-to-nine hours of sleep as the proper amount, to live a life of not feeling tired due to lack of sleep. But even if one gets the proper amount of sleep in one night, it needs to be a habit, not a rare occasion. I am talking about seven-to-nine hours of sleep per night for a minimum of 66 days, before we rule out the lack of sleep as an issue.

Why 66 days? According to a 2009 study performed by researchers from University College London, it takes an average of 66 days to get a new habit to stick. It varies from individual to individual, of course, but 66 was the average. Remember this number as you continue to work to improve different areas of your life. Don't quit or give up. You are worth the time and effort. Remember that persistence is one of the greatest keys to success.

Moving forward. **Subluxation or fixation of our joints causes neurological inhibition, or short circuits within the nervous system, which lead to dysfunction, which lead to soreness and pain, which then lead to degeneration and decay**. During this degenerative process, there are many warning signs or symptoms, just like the gauges on a car telling us something is wrong.

Let me paint a picture of a common situation I've seen in my office. For example, let's discuss a sore neck. I often hear, "I guess I just slept wrong." Someone goes to bed at night feeling great, and they wake up in the morning, and suddenly they can barely turn their head. They do a quick search on Google, find someone with good reviews, and then the call comes in. They come in, fill out a new patient application, then we review their history with them…

…and wow, it is amazing that some people are still alive after the things they have been through. Needless to say, there's usually a lot more to it than a simple "I guess I just slept wrong."

People have all kinds of injuries in their past. There is the motorcycle accident, the high school football trauma, the crutches for three months after a knee injury, the history of the broken collar bone (clavicle), the on-again-off-again pounding headaches over the last 14 months which the patient has been self-medicating for with over the counter medications… and of course, the wrist sprain that happened five years ago when the patient performed a back hand spring with a double twist during a BBQ at their friend's house over the fourth of July weekend, and oops, the trampoline broke.

This is just a small sample of some things that come up during a brief history of the patient's life. So, to answer the question, "Why am I having this neck pain?" **You are having these symptoms because your body is letting you know something is wrong! Isn't that fantastic? We all have a built-in warning system with multiple levels of warning signs, from feeling tired to experiencing sharp, throbbing head and neck pain. All of these signals exist to let us know that something is** not right within us. To solve the issue, we must look at our chemical, structural, and emotional makeup to see what we have been neglecting, or where we've been overindulging.

We have all heard of muscle memory. Look at a basketball player who can make amazing throws and catches or a tennis player who can make shots that seem impossible. These amazing players usually have something in common and that is practice, practice, and practice. Muscle memory works both in the positive way we would normally think of it but it also works the other way. If you have a sprained ankle and end up on crutches for a period of time, your body has now learned muscle behavior patterns such as a shorter stride and possible tilted pelvis to accommodate a boot or brace which you wore to help and protect the injured area. These patterns can be hard to break. We all know how difficult it can be to form a new habit: remember the 66 days from above. This is why **the way we receive care after an injury is so important to the physiology of the body**. If we learn a new habit of altering our gait pattern for 4-6 weeks while we heal up from an injury, we need to make sure that when the injury is healed, we then look at the overall function of the associated joints, and how this altered functioning has affected our nervous system. This is something that a thorough exam can check for if done in the detail and fashion that gives more than what is expected.

So many times, X-rays of the spine and pelvis show signs of degeneration and wear. The patient had no idea their back had a lateral curvature called a scoliosis, or a loss of lordosis. But take an X-ray, and there it is, in black, white and gray. This is when the patient begins to understand that even though their pain just started this morning, much of what they are seeing on the X-ray has been there for years yet their pain just started this morning after a supposed restless night of sleep. Patients will often ask, "If the degeneration of the spine was there for the last two-to-three years, why have I not had neck pain sooner than this?" **Why? Because our bodies are amazing and fantastic.** We can have pressure on a nerve causing dysfunction *long* before we may notice pain. Pain is not the initial indication of a problem. **There are small clues that are usually associated with the pain such as tightness, stiffness, tender and palpable muscle fibers, which may go unnoticed by the patient. This is why it is so important to perform daily or close to daily activities such as stretching, and the foam roller, so that we notice even slight changes in our range of motion and increased muscle soreness for seemingly no reason.** It is like checking the gauges on your dash to make sure your fuel tank is not running too low to make your trip, or making sure you are not past the mileage for your oil change or tire rotation.

Symptoms are our body's way of telling us something is wrong. The key here is to train ourselves to recognize these symptoms as early as possible, by performing preventive maintenance systems such as getting seven-to-nine hours of sleep per night, stretching four-to-five days per week, foam rolling four-to-five days per week, exercising four-to-five days per week, drinking 1/2 our body weight in ounces of water every day, eating properly five-to-six days per week, reading daily to rest and stimulate our minds, and so on. Most importantly, we must do all of these things consistently.

Our body's warning system is fantastic, but we must learn the language of our bodies. We must not dumb it down with unneeded medications, whether these are over the counter or prescribed.

Now, I am not one to damn medications. Medications save lives every day. But as a doctor, I can see that medications are also blatantly overutilized and have negative effects on our bodies, much like sugar and artificial sweeteners. We must be careful not to judge those around us about their choices and habits. We must first take a look at ourselves, and lead by example, as we strive to listen to our bodies and not pump them full of sugar when we are tired, or dumb down our nervous system signals and warnings to us by pumping ourselves full of medications every time we feel the first hint of pain.

Have a relationship with your body, know your body like you would want to know those closest to you. Nurture this relationship like you would an important friendship. Encourage communication with your body, with activities both physical and emotional. Listen to the signals of tightness, stiffness, and of tender and palpable muscle fibers. Be consistent in all the good habits that you either have or will establish as you learn more about your amazing human body.

Chapter 2

UNDERSTANDING WHY OUR BODIES HURT.

Every person is an individual who needs to be looked at as an individual. With that being said, we are all human beings, so we all share common traits. I feel confident we can use this as a baseline to begin the conversation as to whether or not you, I, a neighbor, a brother, a coworker, and so on could be helped with chiropractic care.

Let's look at the human body and discuss what the top four things are which are needed for basic human life. Let's think of it as a **Health Pyramid**.

At the base of this pyramid would be food. Without food, a typical human could live for only 30-45 days, so I would say this needs to be included. Going up one level, I would put water. A human can only live 10-15 days without water, so this must also be included. Another level up is oxygen, because without oxygen, we are good for only about three minutes. Granted, someone who is in good shape could *maybe* survive six minutes, but that's not very long.

The top of our pyramid is reserved for the undisputed champion, nerve flow. You can eat an amazing diet, you can drink the purest water, and breathe the cleanest air, but if you stop nerve flow through our bodies — by severing the spinal cord just below the brainstem — then your heart will stop, your intestines will not function, and your body will shut down in a matter of seconds.

Now the good news is that most of us do not have severed spinal cords, but we may have pressure on our cord. We may also have nerve root irritation due to many possible conditions, such as a herniated disc, a bulging disc, facet hypertrophy, osteoarthritis and so on. These are the things chiropractic is so good at helping and preventing.

Clearly, nerve flow throughout our nervous system is of utmost importance to life. If you have subluxations, then you have neurological inhibition. This means your nervous system, which controls every muscle, tissue and organ in your body, is not functioning as well as it could be. This means that you can be helped with chiropractic care.

Now, I cannot speak to how each individual chiropractic office or chiropractor goes about a new patient examination, but I can speak to how I do things in my office, which will give you a baseline understanding of how the process works. I provide a standard of care which needs to be met with a thorough history, hands-on examination, X-rays if indicated, MRI if needed, and if necessary, a referral to an orthopedic surgeon or neurologist for issues which are beyond the scope of chiropractic care. Our office and every other chiropractic office should give you a thorough evaluation and examination, allowing you to be given a baseline of where you are right now, so a plan can be built with you to get you to where you want to be in regards to your health.

What does the new patient exam entail? Well, let me explain. If you are an existing patient of mine, then you have already experienced the system of tests I put each new patient through. Since I began my practice in 2005, I have continued to evolve my practice, through taking courses and trainings.

The first step is a 100-point neurological testing procedure, which I have streamlined over these past 13 years to be very straightforward and simple. Of course, for a patient who has been experiencing chronic pain or severe acute pain, some of these simple movements are more of a challenge to perform. My staff will then take note of these inefficiencies in the nervous system and musculoskeletal system, and we give the new patient a score based on their results, not anyone else's.

From here we will typically order X-rays based on the patient's history and exam findings. In my office, I refer my patients to Valley Radiologists for X-rays, because then, all the films will be read by a radiologist who views films all day, every day. Also, the quality of the films is phenomenal. If we need an MRI or CT, the same facility will already have access to the patient's previous tests. This also gives me access to a network of some amazing physicians throughout the state of Arizona by just picking up the phone.

The more symptoms someone is experiencing, the more important it is for them to get into a chiropractic office and get checked. If you think you may have some deficiencies in your musculoskeletal or nervous system, then get to a chiropractic office and get yourself checked for neurological deficiencies. Find a doctor in your area, or if you're near me, you can just come to our office. Find us at www.PetersWellness.com. There is no need to live in pain. Pain may *be* fantastic, but being *in* pain is not!

Chapter 3

HOW LONG DO I HAVE TO SUFFER WITH THESE SYMPTOMS?

It has been said and I have heard it many times that, "Once you go to a chiropractor, you have to go forever." But this isn't a scary thing. I like to think of going to the chiropractor in the same way I think about going to the gym to do my workouts.

Now, as for me personally, I currently visit the chiropractor once per week, and I work out at the gym five times per week. This is my schedule because I have found that I function extremely well with this regime. Has this always been the case? No. There have been times when I have had to get adjusted three times per week for a time, especially after an injury or setback, after which I get back on track. There have been periods where I worked out six days per week and there have been times when I did not work out for months at a time.

It is my job to recommend the care needed to help each person to function at their best, but it is up to each individual on how they *want* to get there. **The point is that *your* health is yours. It is your body, and you get to choose what you do with and for it.**

As for me, I am motivated by pain and pleasure just like everyone else, and as I get older, I am learning how to be more motivated by pleasure rather than allowing the desire to avoid pain be my motivation. **Surviving is good but thriving is way better.**

There are many factors which help us know what it will take for your body to heal, such as your pain levels, the chronicity of your issues, how you do on your neurological exam, how your X-rays look, your ability to make your scheduled appointments, and also how well you address your emotional, chemical and structural stressors.

In Chiropractic College, we are taught to have the patient complete a Visual Analog Scale (VAS) to rate each area of concern during the initial exam process. If, for instance, you have neck pain, we want to know how you would rate it on a scale of 1-10, with 10 being the worst pain you have ever experienced—for example, pain on the level of child birth, passing of a kidney stone or breaking a bone. This is done for each area of complaint. It is amazing how so many new patients coming in have multiple areas of pain, with scores over a 6 or 7. Many of these patients have been suffering for over five, ten or fifteen years with no resolution at this point.

There are many factors in creating an effective care plan for each individual patient. We must look at the issues that the patient is having and consider the following items.
- When and how was the **Onset** of the patient's issues?
- What makes the pain **Palliative or Provocative** (better or worse)?
- What is the **Quality** of the pain (sharp, dull, achy, burning...)?
- Does the pain **Radiate** or travel and if it does what is the path it takes and when does it do this?
- What is the **Severity** of the pain on a Visual Analog Scale (VAS)?
- Is the **Timing** of the issue constant, frequent or rarely an issue?

The above scale is referred to as the **OPQRST,** and it is a great way to access the problems or issues on a subjective level. It is also a great opportunity to get as much input as possible from the patient.

Imagine someone who describes the following: *"I was at a stoplight in my small compact car about a week ago, and a massive SUV traveling between 30 and 50 mph smashed into the back of my little car, blowing out the back window and putting his bumper practically into my back seat. After I was taken to the hospital for X-rays and a CT Scan, I was released with muscle relaxers and heating and icing instructions. I was told to follow up with my primary care provider (PCP) if issues persisted. My neck is killing me and every time I look up or down the pain goes down, my left arm causing my entire hand to go numb for about 10 minutes. If I try to turn my head to the left or right, I do not get the numbness in my hand, but I get intense sharp pain in my neck on the left side. When I do not move my head, my neck is still constantly sore and it causes my head to pound and my shoulders feel tight and sore. My pain is a 10 out of 10 on the Visual Analog Scale (VAS) and as I stated the pain is constant, but it becomes much worse with certain movements."*

Now, compare the above example to someone who says, "my neck pain is a 2 out of 10 (VAS) after sleeping in a funny position the other night."

These two people will not take the same amount of care to get them out of pain and into full recovery.

Next it is time to review the objective tests which were completed at the initial exam, and review results from other tests the patient had performed at other offices or labs such as blood work, CT or MRI results. I review the patient's score from the initial exam they had in our office. The patient performs 100 specific tests and I look at how many of these they failed during the exam. This is one component used to calculate how many visits and what period of time will be required to get this patient to a point in care where they not only feel the issue has been resolved, but they also feel they have their life back. We also know this objectively because the patient's neurological tests have improved to a point of acceptability.

The next component is usually X-ray results. I don't want to get into a full radiology course here, but I do want to help people better understand X-rays, so that they are not so scary or mysterious. Remember the old saying, "a picture is worth a thousand words?" Before we jump into that, let's discuss some of the basic concepts to help guide you through this next section:

- Anterior (front of the body)
- Posterior (back of the body)
- Lateral (side view)
- A/P View (Anterior to Posterior view or Front to Back view)
- Cervical Spine (neck)
- Thoracic spine (upper and mid-back combined)
- Lumbar spine (lower back)
- Pelvis (hip and tail bone area)
- Lordosis - looking at the spine from the side, this is the curve from the front to the back of the body and is measured **in both the cervical and lumbar portions of the spine and is a necessary part for optimal spinal health.**
- Kyphosis - looking at the spine from the side, this is the curve from the front to the back of the body and is measured **in the thoracic portion of the spine and is a necessary part of optimal spinal health.**
- Scoliosis - this is looking at the spine from the front or the back of the body and it is a curvature that goes side-to-side or laterally. **This is looked for in the**

cervical, thoracic and lumbar portions of the spine and this is a curvature which you do not want to have.

Cervical Spine

For our review of X-rays let's start at the top and work our way down the same way our neurological process operates.

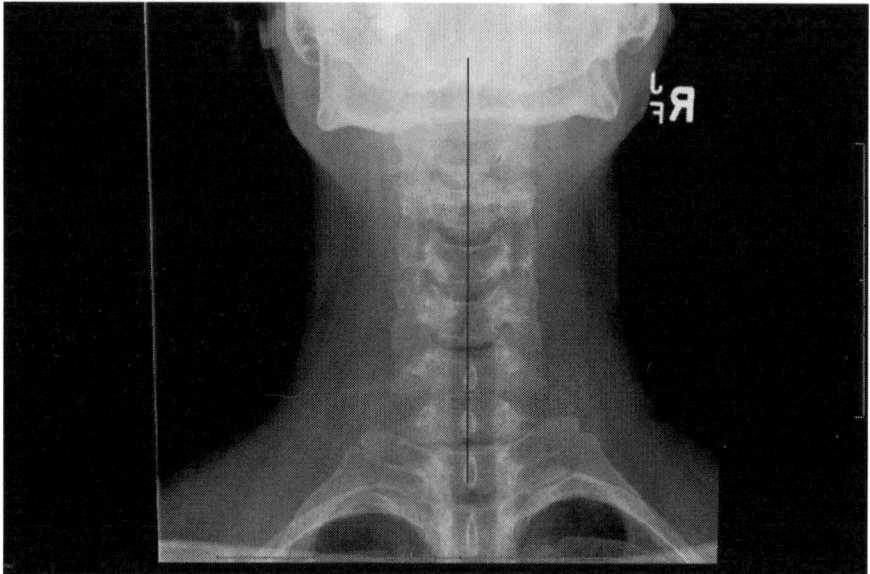

Figure #1 Above: Here we see an example of a posterior to anterior view of the cervical spine. This example is an excellent looking cervical spine from back to front, and I use it as my "normal" example to compare to other X-rays in our office. Notice the black line and how it travels straight down the spine with the spine not deviating from it. This view should not have any lateral (side to side) curves.

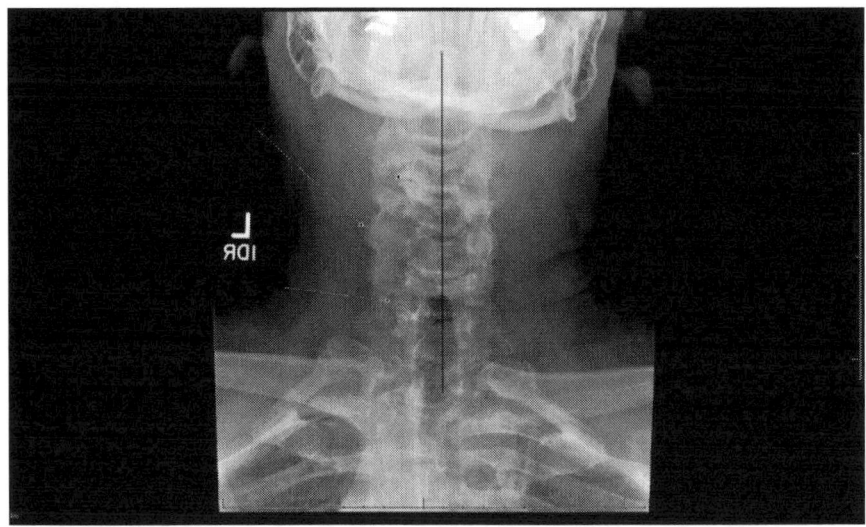

Figure #2 Above: Here we see the back-to-front view of a cervical spine, but now, we see how it looks with degeneration of the facet joints, especially on the left side. Notice there really is not much of a side-to-side or lateral curvature of the spine, but yet we still see Phase 2 Degeneration. This can be caused by Subluxations of the facet joints. Facet joints are the joints that allow movement between a pair of vertebras. If the joints of the spine are locked up and not moving properly, physiological processes begin and early Degenerative Joint Disease (DJD) begins leading to Degenerative Disc Disease (DDD). This X-ray is a perfect example of someone who complains of a stiff neck on and off over time, and never seems to have much of a mechanism of injury except maybe "I slept wrong," or "lots of screen time."

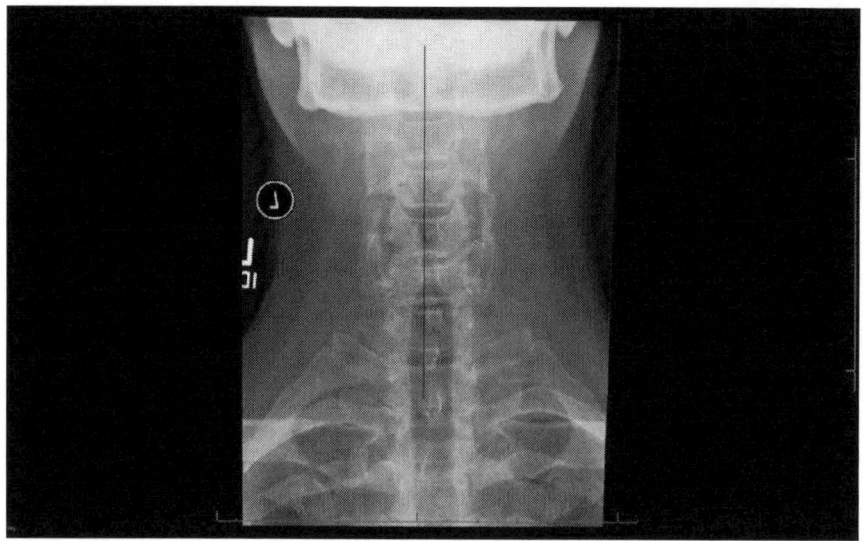

Figure #3 Above: Here is another example of Degenerative Joint Disease (DJD) and Degenerative Disc Disease (DDD). Compare this to Figure #2, where the degeneration was much more widespread. This is an example of why early signs of degeneration should not be ignored. Remember it is your health and your choice. Understand, if you choose to ignore early signs of degeneration it means that late signs of degeneration will come sooner than they need to.

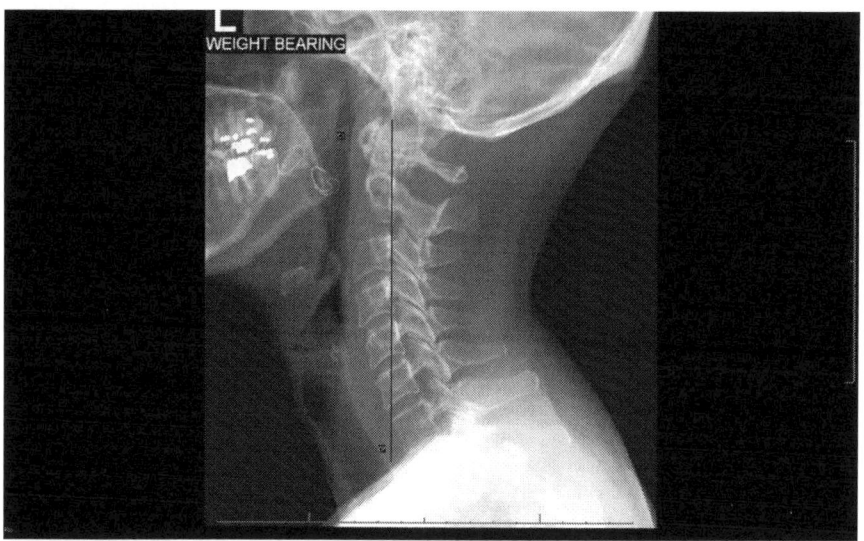

Figure #4 Above: Normal Cervical Lordosis:

The most common issue I see in the cervical spine is the loss of the lordotic curve (see figure #5). This issue can be absolutely detrimental to nerve flow traveling through the neck and out to the entire body. This loss of lordotic curvature can lead to an obvious anterior head posture which increases the amount of pressure and strain on the cervical spine musculature and joints of the bones of the spine called vertebras.

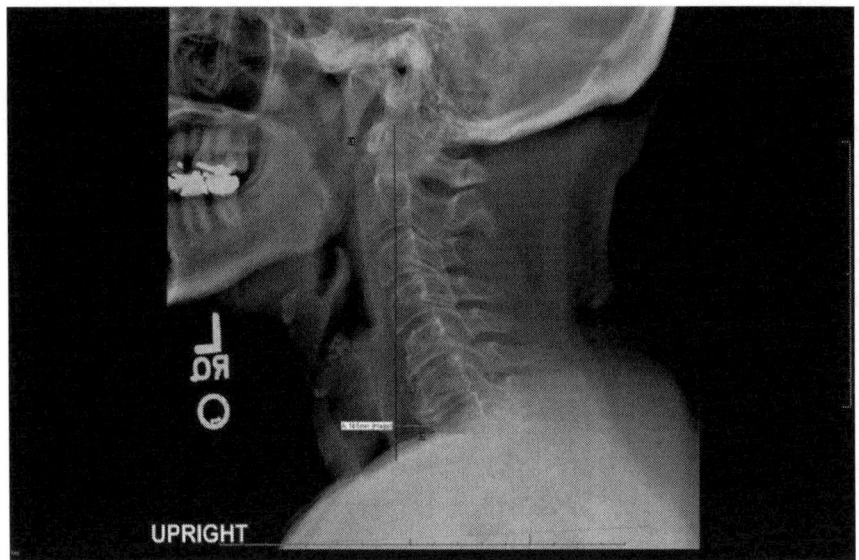

Figure #5 Above: Loss of the Cervical Lordosis: Notice the black line (cervical gravity line) dropped from the center of the dens of C2. This line should drop down on the anterior two thirds of the C7 Vertebral Body. Instead this line drops down in front of or anterior to the C7 Vertebral Body. There is almost a complete loss of the cervical lordosis and by this, I mean there is no anterior to posterior curvature in the cervical spine compared to our normal cervical lordotic curvature in figure #4.

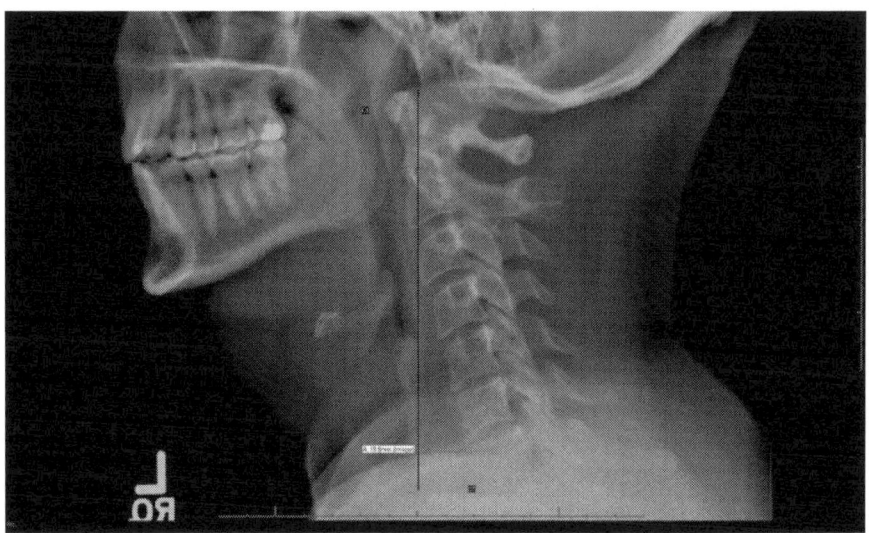

Figure #6 Above: Loss of the Cervical Lordosis with beginning phases of Degenerative Joint Disease and Degenerative Disc Disease.

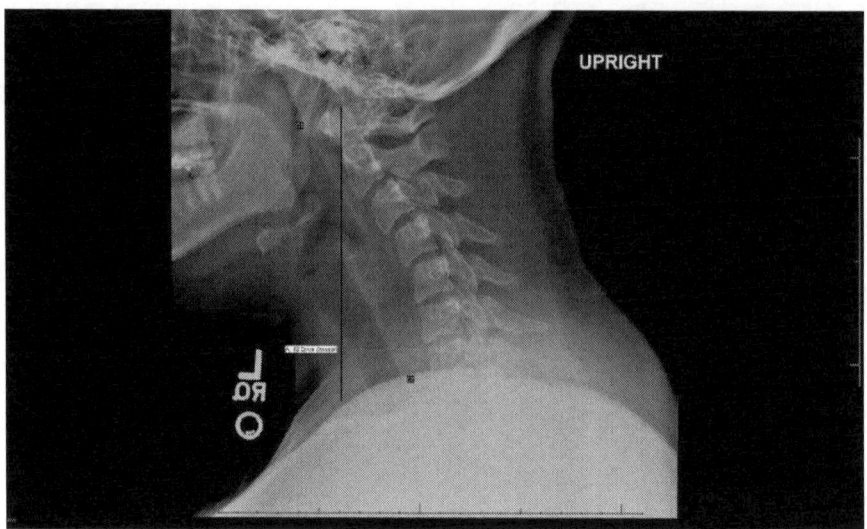

Figure #7 Above: Loss of Cervical Lordosis along with actual reversal of the cervical lordosis. Remember all of these X-rays were taken with the patient positioned by the X-ray Technician in what *should* be normal alignment, but as you can see, it is amazing what we can hide under our flesh.

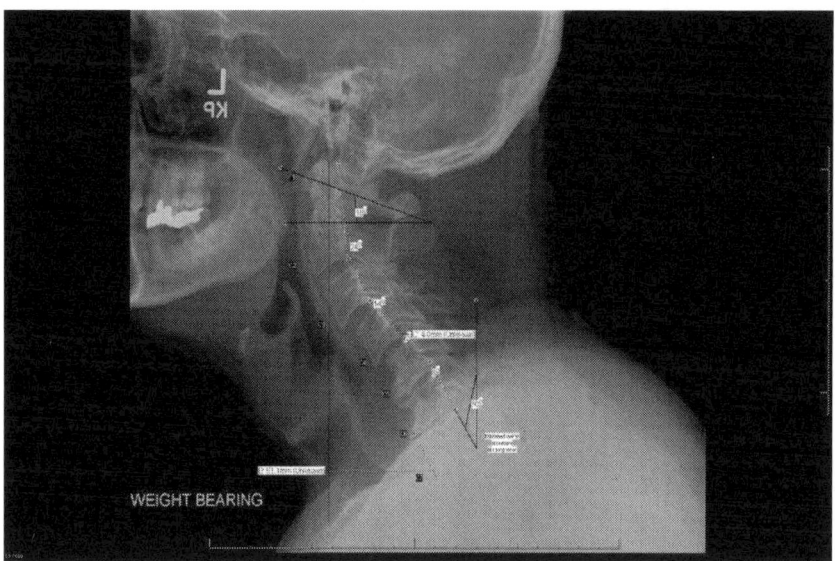

Figure #8 Above: Loss of Cervical Lordosis left untreated. By now, you should be able to tell that this is a *very* degenerated cervical spine. When I see a spine like this, I shudder at the way this person must suffer needlessly. If only he had begun chiropractic care, and stuck with it from an earlier age. I can still help this patient, but physical matter does have its limits.

Thoracic Spine

Now let's take a look at the lateral or side-to-side curvatures of the Thoracic Spine which come off of the midline of the body when looking at the patient from front to back or back to front. These curves are called scoliotic curvatures and there should not be any of these. If there is, it usually requires extra time to get the nervous system functioning at its best due to the physiological strain these scoliotic curves cause on the musculoskeletal system. First, let's take a look at a normal A-P or P-A Thoracic View.

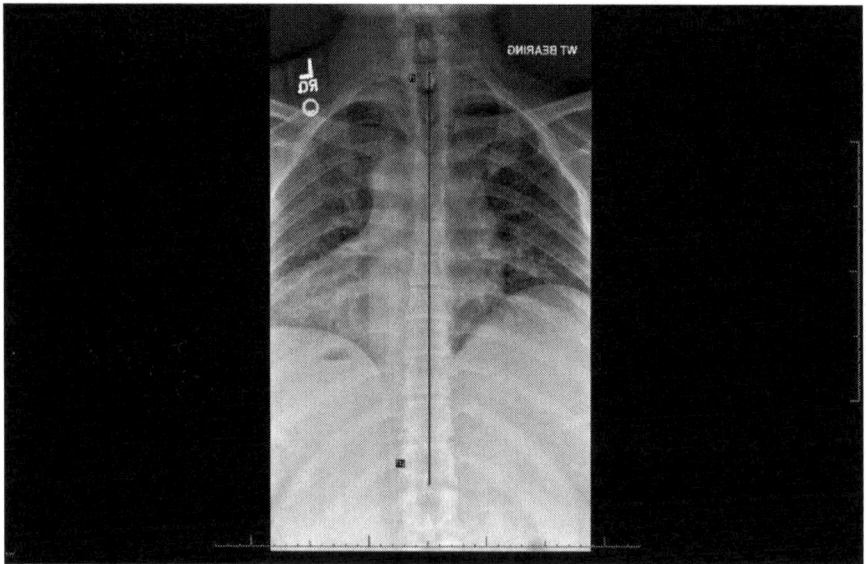

Figure #9 Above: Do you notice how the black line stays on the middle of the posterior portion of the vertebral bodies? This is a great looking spine with no sign of scoliosis.

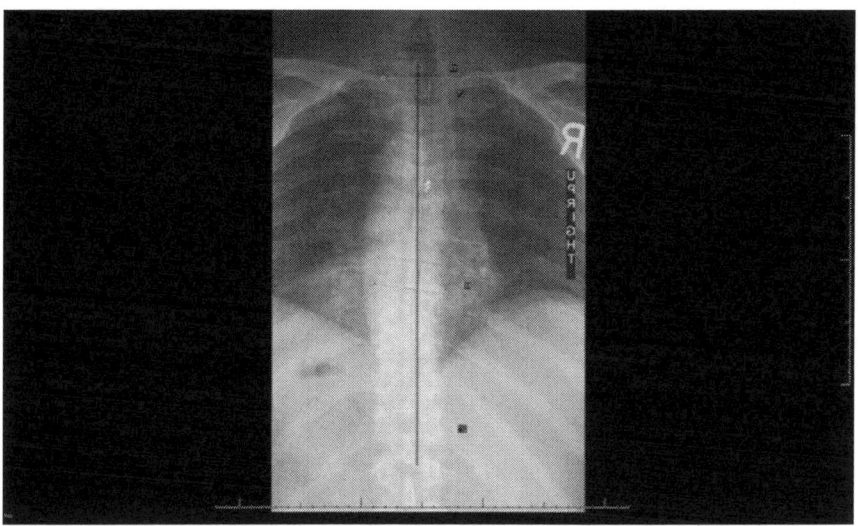

Figure #10 Above: The above photo shows an 8-degree levorotatory scoliosis. You can see how the spine goes left of the black line

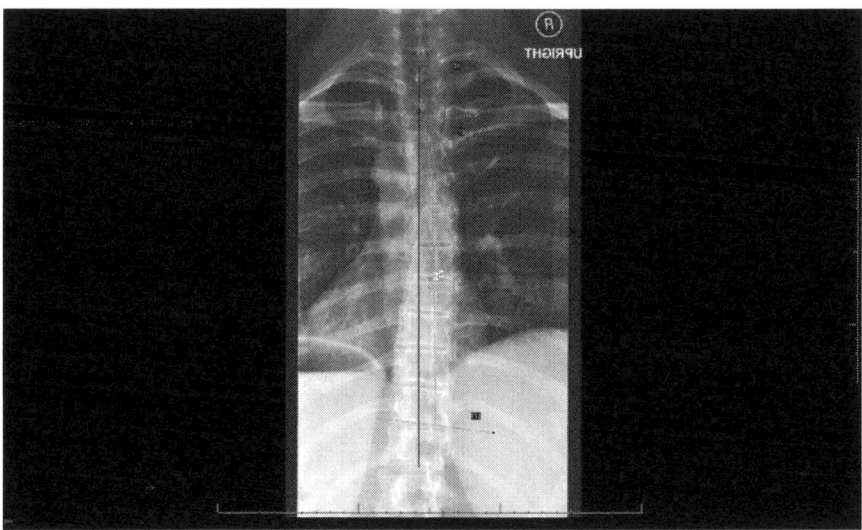

Figure #11 Above: The above photo shows a 14-degree dextrorotatory scoliosis. You can see how the spine goes right of the black line.

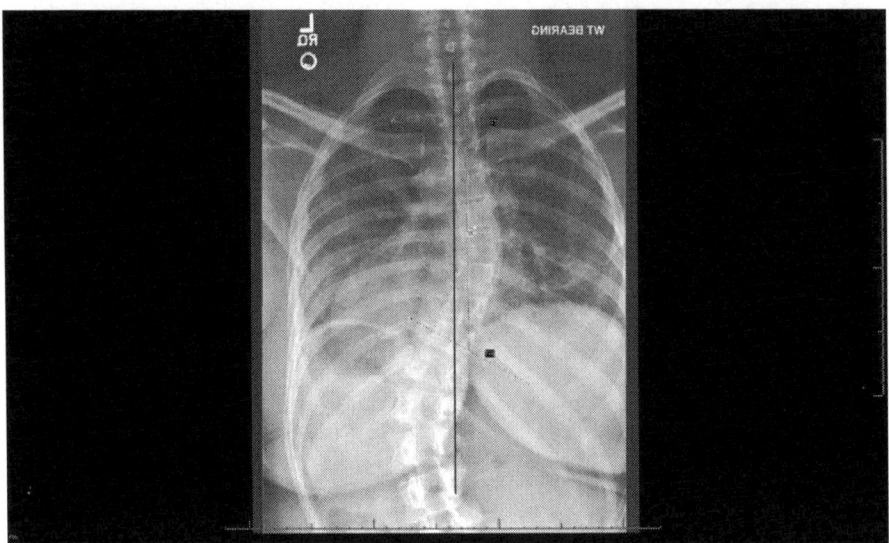

Figure #12 Above: The above photo shows a 38-degree dextrorotatory scoliosis.

It is important to note that if you have been told that you have a certain degree of scoliosis in your spine, that you also be told the beginning and ending points from where the curve was measured. In some instances, if the scoliosis is not measured from the same places in the spine as it was originally, the measurement could change by quite a bit. This would have you believe your curve is getting better or worse, when in all actuality, it was simply measured from different points.

A scoliotic curvature can also be found in the neck (cervical spine) and the low back (lumbar spine).

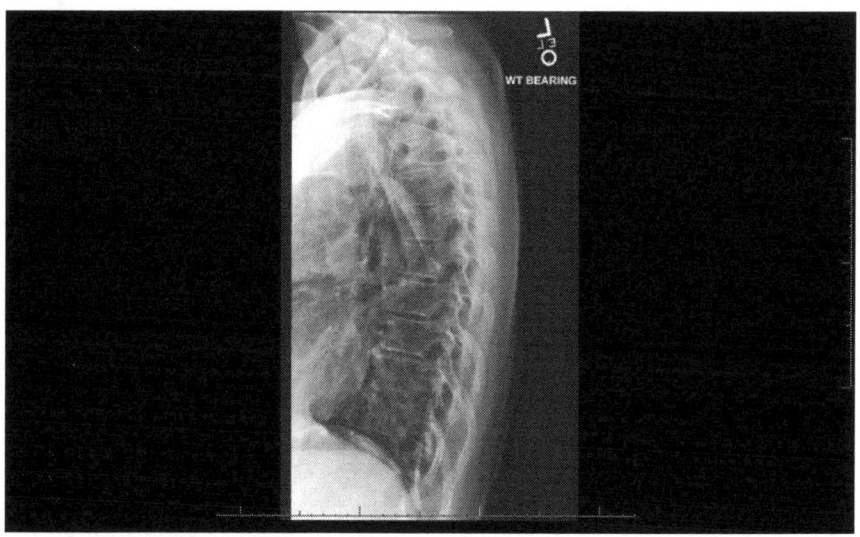

Figure #13 Above: This is an example of a normal Lateral Thoracic X-ray.

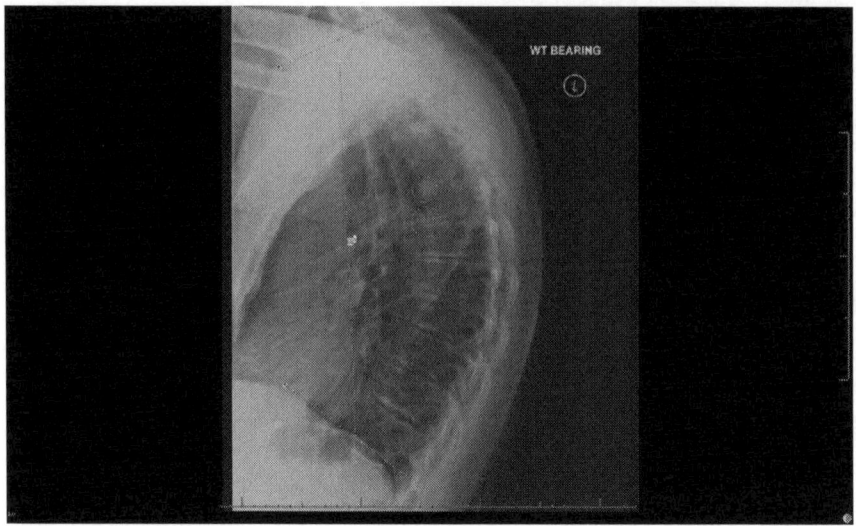

Figure #14 Above: This is an example of a hyperkyphotic thoracic spine with evidence of osteophytes and hypertrophy of some of the superior and inferior endplates of the mid-thoracic spine. The osteophytes are bone growth responses to improper pressure and restriction of movement left unchecked by regular chiropractic care.

Lumbar Spine

The lumbar spine or the lower back is an area where so many people are debilitated by chronic pain and disability. The lumbar spine just like the cervical and thoracic spine should be straight up and down on the A-P or P-A view. There should be no side-to-side deviation (known as a scoliosis).

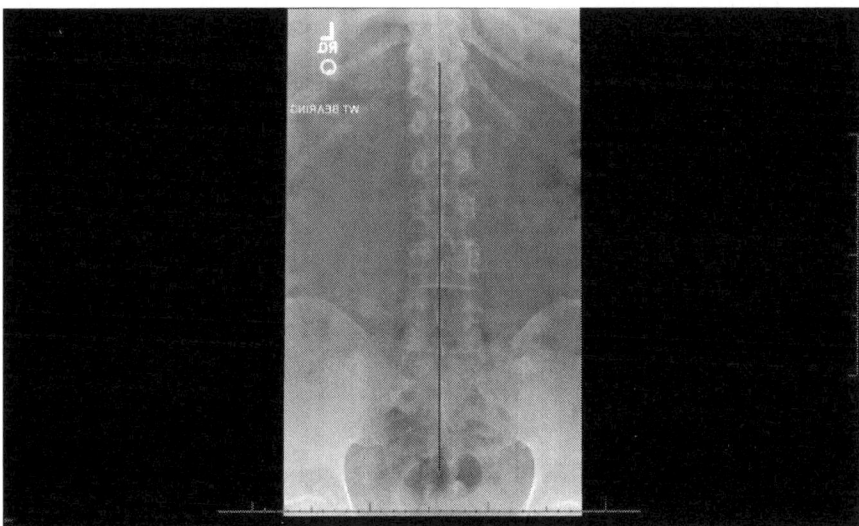

Figure #15 Above: Sample AP Lumbar. This is an example of a properly aligned A-P or P-A view of the lumbar spine or low back.

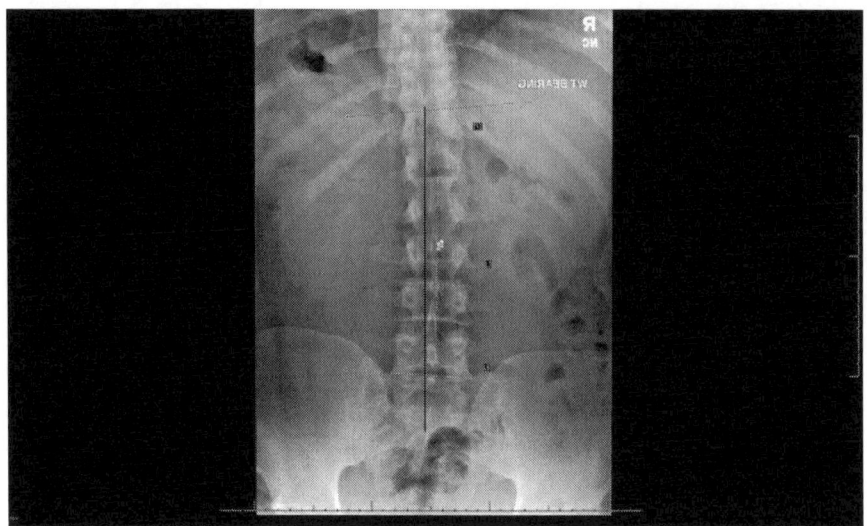

Figure #16 Above: Here we see an 8-degree dextrorotatory scoliosis of the lumbar spine measured from T12 to S1. Notice the deviation of the spine from the black line.

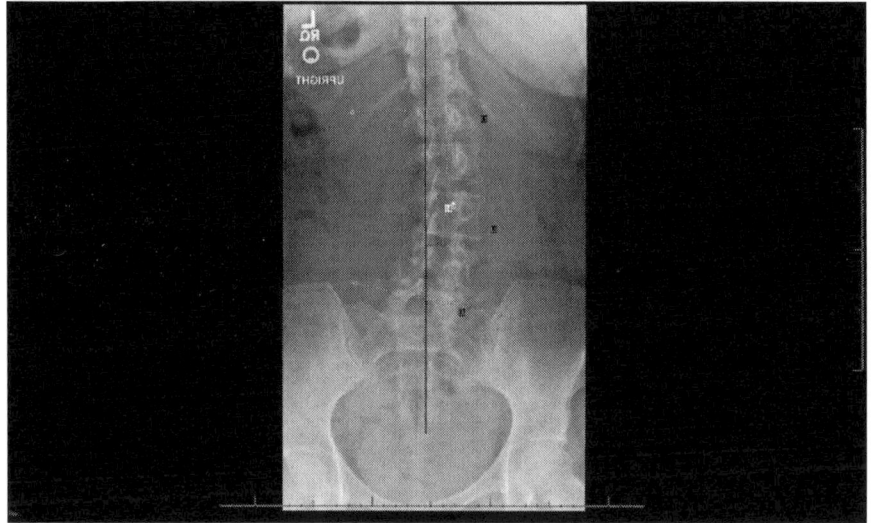

Figure #17 Above: Here we see a 16-degree Levorotatory Scoliosis measured from L1-S1.

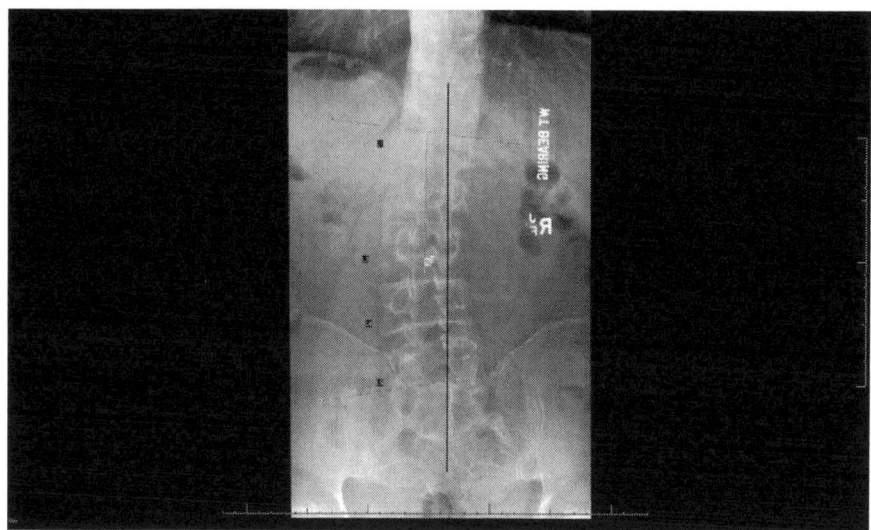

Figure #18 Above: Here we see a 14-degree dextrorotatory scoliosis of the lumbar spine measured from L1-L5. Notice the deviation of the spine from the black line.

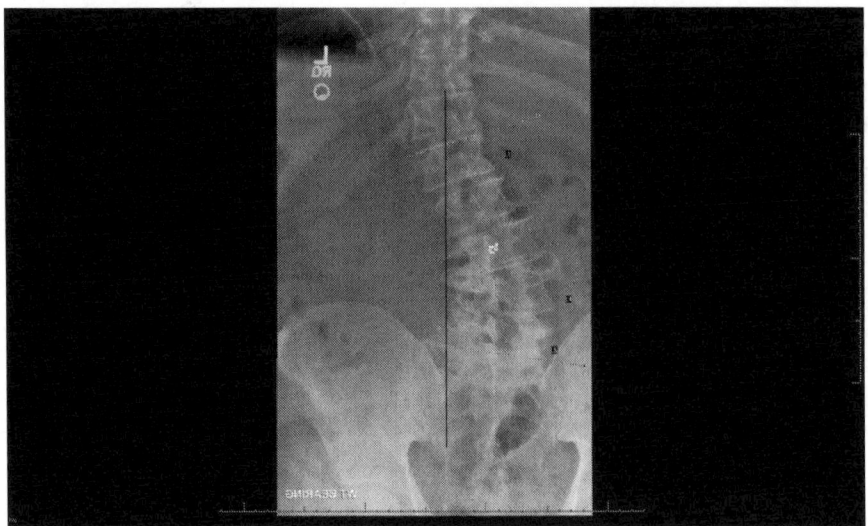

Figure #19 Above: Here we see a 24-degree scoliosis with evidence of its chronicity due to the large osteophytes and syndesmophytes coming off of the vertebres. This degeneration, pictured above, is what everyone talks about when they refer to Degenerative Joint Disease (DJD) and Degenerative Disc Disease (DDD).

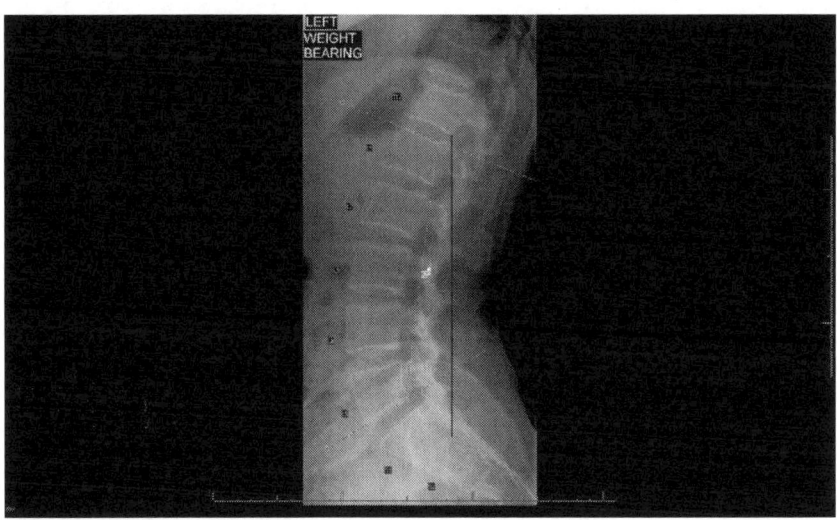

Figure #20 Above: The above photo shows a nice looking (within normal limits) lumbar lordosis. A normal lordosis measures between 50-60 degrees from the superior endplate of L1 to the inferior endplate of L5.

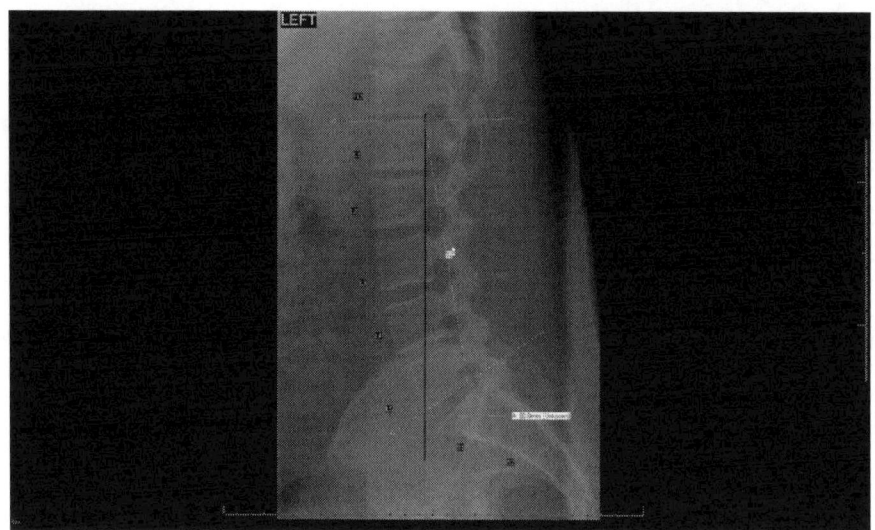

Figure #21 Above: The above photo shows a lumbar spine with about 50% loss of lordosis.

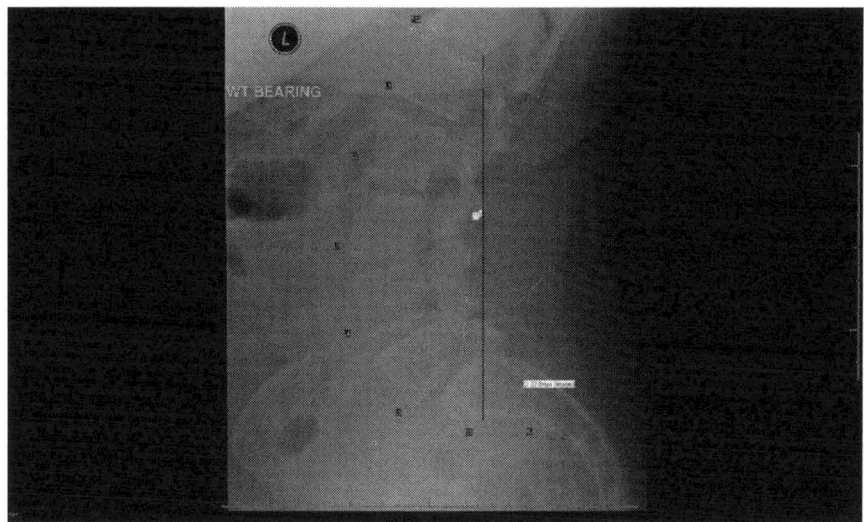

Figure #22 Above: The above photo shows a lumbar lordosis with, as you can see, too much of a lordosis.

Normal is between 50 degrees and 60 degrees, while this one measures 74 degrees.

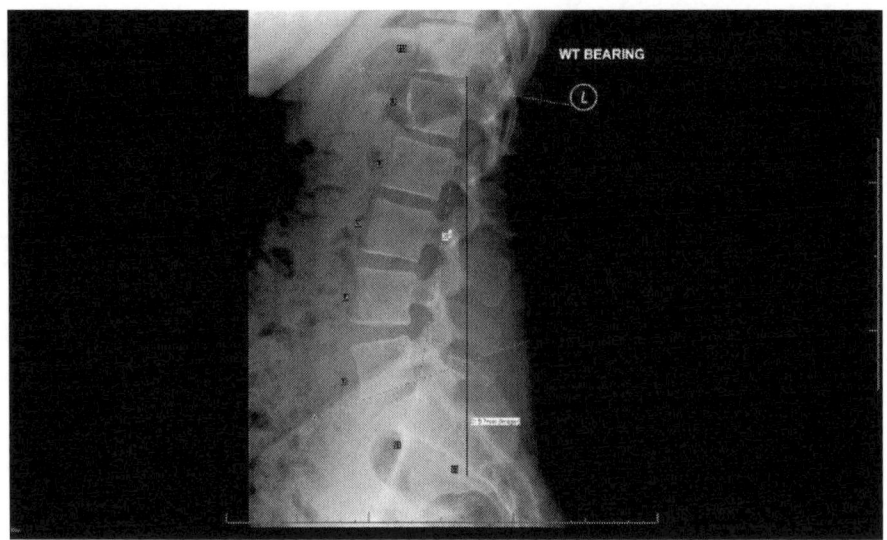

Figure #23 Above: The above photo is a lateral lumbar with loss of lordosis but notice the 60.8mm of anterior translation.

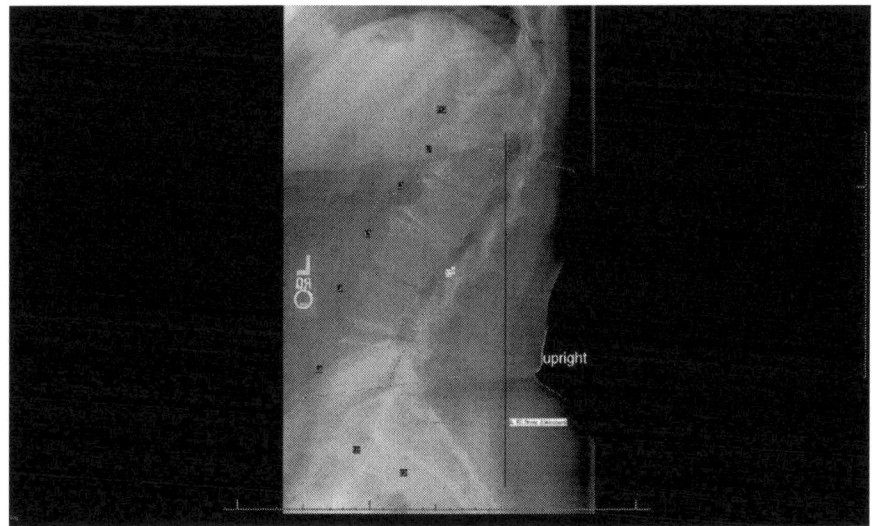

Figure #24 Above: The above photo has a severe amount of posterior translation measuring 57.8mm the opposite of the anterior translation photo. Both of these patients began with severe lower back pain but both were immensely helped with chiropractic and home traction.

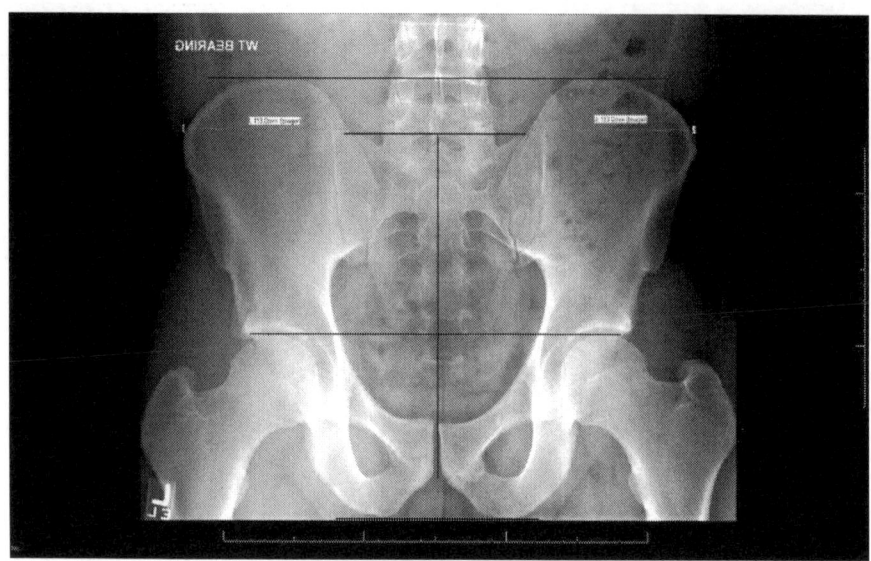

Figure #25 Above: The above figure is an AP Pelvic X-ray and is an example of a well-balanced pelvis.

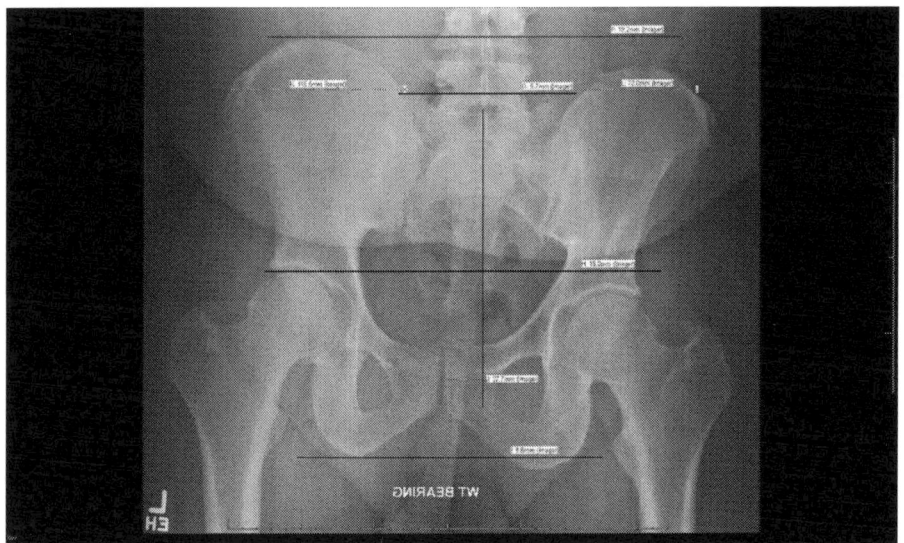

Figure #26 Above: The above figure is an example of an AP Pelvic X-ray with a high left iliac crest (crest of the ilium).

Once the pain levels, objective neurological tests and X-rays are reviewed then it is time to look at the activities of daily living, and how the patient's life is being impacted due to the issues they are experiencing. If the patient's symptoms are so severe that they are having difficulties bathing and dressing themselves, then obviously the visit frequency will be greater in the beginning, due to the severity of the presenting symptoms.

In most cases, the patient should have quite a bit of relief within the first two weeks of care. By the end of the first month, they should be able to see a 50% improvement in the re-performance of all the tests which were performed on day one. So, if a new patient failed 40 tests out of 100 on the first visit, then we expect to see them fail only 20 tests or less next time. This means they have gone from a 60% success rate to an 80% success rate. Our goal for patients is to have them scoring at 85% or higher, failing only 15% or less.

With the above outline and description, it can now be understood why a care plan could be anywhere from four weeks to twelve months. People will ask me how long will it take for their back pain to go away, and it really varies depending on the individual. This question is easily answered, but only after a thorough history, examination and X-rays with possible MRI or CT scans have been performed. Only after we have a more thorough understanding of the specific patient and their underlying conditions, can we understand the specific steps and time needed for the healing process.

Chapter 4

WHAT IS YOUR HEALTH WORTH?

With what is happening in the area of health insurance, as well as government involvement in almost every direction we turn, the cost of health care is on the rise. In 2016, many patients saw their deductibles triple, as their co-pays increased by 10% - 50%. As all of this happened, the costs of their monthly insurance premiums tripled as well.

Now, many people may not have even noticed this, but the company they work for may have absorbed the increasing cost of health insurance. But successful companies are not stupid. If the overhead increases, they'll find another area to cut costs and expenses, and this will trickle down into increased product and service prices for us, the consumers. This means that we are the ones who will take yet another hit to our pocket books.

In the end, it is always more intelligent to invest in *yourself,* by focusing on improving your time, energy, money, education (formal or informal), exercise and proper eating.

Notice this encompasses the emotional, structural and chemical components of your health. It covers your investing in yourself and your future health. What could be better than that?

Even today, many people still do not have insurance, or their deductible is so high that unless they end up on life support, their so-called "health insurance" will not benefit them except in a life-threatening situation.

The cost of chiropractic care varies tremendously depending on whether you have insurance or not. What many people may not realize is that there are a lot of technicalities involved with how the process works. If you have insurance, then your doctor will check to see if their office is contracted with that particular insurance company. Then they must look at whether you have a deductible or not. Deductibles can vary from $250 to as much as $10,000. If your care is going to go towards your deductible, then the provider must use the contracted rates with the insurance company, and you are responsible for your insurance plan's deductible amount. **Once the deductible is met, if you have one, then the provider must look to what your plans "co-pay" or "coinsurance amount" is.** This amount can vary from zero dollars to $75, depending on your specific insurance plan.

Now, if you do *not* have insurance, then the providers office will still have the normal fees, but just like being contracted with your insurance company, your provider can reduce those fees if you are on a self-pay plan. This will allow them to do the same thing in regards to matching something closer to the insurance rate.

Along with health insurance and cash plans, our office also handles a lot of personal injury cases. Personal Injury Cases or Auto Accident Cases are handled by the patient filling out a lien, and the lien is then applied to the patient, until the bill gets paid from the insurance company. Then, once the balance is paid off, the lien is released. Cost for personal injury is very different from other insurance or cash care because there are no contracted rates and mostly because payment may not be received for two-to-three years after the care is completed. There is also a chance of your provider having to testify in the case; speaking from personal experience, I have done this before, but only once at the time of this writing. The key to a great defense for the patient is to have fantastic notes which document the patient's care in great detail so there is no doubt in the minds of the jurors that the care was needed and that there was suffering and inconvenience to the patient due to the injuries they received from the accident.

One thing regarding cost of health care is the misconception of *actual* "Health Care" versus what I'd prefer to call "Sick Care."

True, actual Health Care is getting the proper amount of sleep, drinking the proper amount of water, using the foam roller, exercising, proper eating, and taking care of our emotional needs on a consistent basis. All of the things I just mentioned cost very little compared to Sick Care.

Sick Care, which is what is generally called "health care," is what our insurance plans were meant to cover. Broken bones, heart attacks, cancer, leukemia, and other horrible ailments which plague our society are what Sick Care (AKA, our Health Care Plans) were meant for.

Think of it this way. Should our auto insurance cover oil changes, rotation of tires, and tune ups? No, because these are not the responsibility of the insurance companies. These are the responsibility of the vehicle owners. Sure, some items may be under a particular warranty. But when it comes to our bodies, they might have no warranty, but they *do* have an amazing self-healing ability which is controlled by our nervous system.

So, what is the value of caring for this master control system? Some would say it's priceless. As for me, I prefer to put some type of monetary value on things, and for our office those prices are covered up front. That way, we give the patient the freedom to decide what things are more important than their health, and to hopefully make better choices regarding their health now and in the future.

It comes down to this. We must all invest time, energy, and money into the things we love. The real question is: how much do you love your health?

Chapter 5

ISN'T MY PROBLEM JUST TIGHT MUSCLES?

Back when I lived in California, I was a certified massage therapist. Massage therapy, or myofascial release, has fantastic benefits for the human body. This background experience with massage is the reason why we have massage therapy in our office. Some insurance companies with specific plans still cover myofascial release, or massage, and we will check a patient's insurance plan and let them know if they can have this done as part of care under their insurance. For some people, there is currently no additional cost for adding a massage to their visit. For others, there is an additional co-pay, and we let them know what their insurance requires them to pay for this service.

So, let's talk about muscles. There are different reasons why muscles get tight in the first place. For example, muscles can get tight and sore after an intense workout. Most people have experienced this. If you search for tight muscles online you will likely find the term Delayed Onset Muscle Soreness.

When people go to the gym, they will often focus on one set of muscles at a time, for instance, the legs. Those of you who've experienced a "leg day" understand how a heavy workout can make muscles feel sore. Many people do not enjoy working out their legs, because it can be very tiring. But then, when they finally work on their legs, they do the leg workout extra heavy, because they know they do not do legs enough. This has a dramatic effect. Within the next 24 hours they can barely walk or get up from a chair. In this case, the muscle tightness is due more to the fact that they spent so long not working out their legs, as opposed to the intense workout itself. **Also, in this case, the muscle tightness and soreness is a good sign. It helps us recognize that we have not been working our legs enough, and we may want to put more focus into working that part of our bodies. So yes, more "leg days" are necessary.**

When muscles are kept in a shortened position, they tend to get very tight, whereas muscles kept in a stretched position for long periods of time tend to become weakened. A prime example of this is sitting.

Now I know some of us are up and moving all day, and rarely sit for more than 10 minutes at a time. But then there are many of us who have desk jobs, and sit for very long periods of time. Think about it: I have patients that drive an hour or more to work, and then another hour or more to drive home at the end of the day. In the middle of this is an eight-to-ten-hour work day. After that they may go home and have dinner while sitting at the kitchen counter or kitchen table, and if there is any energy left, they probably just sit in front of the television or computer for some mindless activity after a very long day.

The key here is that the *action* of sitting, (yes, I write the word *action,* because there are muscles being activated during the sitting process) causes certain muscles of the core to be in a shortened position for long periods at a time, and this causes these muscles to become tightened. This is why those big Swiss Exercise Balls are so awesome for laying on your back as you stretch your abdominal muscles. Our hip flexors and pectoralis muscles also tend to get very tight in the sitting position. The foam roller is extremely valuable for loosening and stretching these muscles.

I am not saying that stretching is the best thing you can do for tight muscles, but it definitely ranks in the top three. Along with chiropractic adjustments, the foam roller, yoga, palates and massage, stretching is an absolute essential element to feeling awesome, living to your fullest potential and not suffering with tight muscles.

Since we've discussed tight muscles, we also have to discuss inhibited muscles. Broadening that further, let's discuss weak muscles versus neurologically inhibited muscles. You may be thinking there is really no difference, but this is not the case. A muscle can be taut, tight and tender, yet still be capable of firing as long as the electrical signal from the brain down the spinal cord (and then out to the muscle) is not being interfered with.

But if the nerve flow is interrupted, even the strongest and largest muscles will be unable to fire and function due to the lack of nerve flow to that muscle. Think of going into a room and flipping the light switch, but the lights stay off. You find the electrical control panel, open it up, find the tripped breaker and flip it, go back to the room and like magic the lights are now working when the light switch is flipped to the "on" position.

Let's look at another example of an electrical system to help us understand a muscle which is neurologically inhibited. First, what does it mean for a muscle to be neurologically inhibited?

Think of the power source to the muscle being blocked by some type of short circuit. Let's use the analogy of a tripped breaker in a simple hair dryer as an example. Hairdryers have a built-in circuit breaker on the power cord. This design, as we all know, is to protect someone from being electrocuted. The setup is very nice because on the end of the plug there is usually a red button and a black button. One button allows you to see when the breaker is tripped and the other is to reset the breaker and reconnect the circuit. Now a key insight here is if the hairdryer electrical components are still wet, the breaker will not hold the reset and when you plug the cord in, the breaker will immediately trip, and you will have to wait until the electrical components have dried out so the moisture does not cause another short circuit. Once the internal components of the hairdryer have dried off, and as long as the moisture has not done permanent damage, you can now reset the circuit breaker and begin to use the hairdryer again.

Now let's correlate the above analogy to the human body. Let's pick one muscle to use as our example: say, the triceps brachii, which runs down the back of the arm. I am picking this muscle because most people are familiar with it.

The triceps brachii's job is to extend the elbow and the long head assists in adduction and extension of the shoulder.

The innervation to the triceps brachii is a combination of C6, C7, C8 and T1 (this is the lower part of the neck and the first segment of the upper back) and the nerve name is the radial nerve. If this muscle tests weak (or is inhibited), it could mean many things.

Just as with the hairdryer, the first thing we want to check is the power source. The power source for the triceps brachii is the area of the lower neck referred to as C6, C7, C8 and T1. These nerve roots can be impinged upon due to facet joint fixation, disc bulge, tight muscles, bone spurs or some type of space occupying lesion at the spinal level.

The treacherous path the nerve takes from the lower part of the neck can also give opportunity for entrapment, as it travels along the neck to the upper arm. This is why it is also important to check all the joints which the nerve passes over. This means we must check the shoulder complex including the clavicle, scapula and humerus then we must check the elbow area including this time the distal end of the humerus and the radius and ulna. Once all the involved joints are checked, then we must check the muscles around each and every joint involved.

The logical order to follow, if we want to determine the possible causes, depends upon the history of the patient. If the patient was hit with a baseball bat on the back of the arm, the approach would be different than if the patient came in complaining of neck pain and headaches which came on gradually.

For an example of another electrical system, think of a desktop computer. If you sat down to use the computer and you turned on the monitor and hit the power button but nothing happened, what would you do? Well, over the years, I have learned from my amazing IT guy, Les Jorgensen, that if you are having an issue with your computer try rebooting it, after you make sure it is plugged in and has power.

I mean really, what is the purpose of going through all the stress and irritation of having a computer problem which merely ends up being a tripped breaker? Then there are all the times that the computer was acting up one way or another, and a simple quick reboot got rid of the incredible irritation.

Think about it: a simple reset and things just get better. Always, always, always, when it comes to your computer, start with the power source. When it comes to the human body, do the same thing.

Our spinal cord is simply a continuation of the brain. The nerves which extend from the spinal cord and travel throughout the body are also a continuation of the brain, much like the wires running through your home are a continuation of the electrical system of your home.

If the nerve supply to muscles, tissues or organs is being interfered with, then none of these will function as well as they should. So, if a patient is complaining of lower back pain, it makes sense to check all the muscles around the pelvis and lower back. This will allow us to find out what is working, and what is not.

One might check the hamstrings and find them neurologically inhibited, meaning when they are isolated, and when tested, they do not fire properly. This does not necessarily mean the muscles are physically weak or injured. It could be that the nerve which activates them is not sending its signal properly due to nerve impingement from many possible causes such as soft tissue pressure from a bulging or herniated disc, facet joint fixation or it could be something as bad as a space-occupying lesion such as a metastatic or non-metastatic tumor.

On the other hand, it may be a sprain or strain to muscle or tendon itself or something more severe such as a tear. It could also be an old injury which has led to tendonitis, bursitis, or muscle inflammation.

If it was quick and easy, over-the-counter medications for pain would not be such a hot commodity. Sometimes, taking a pill to block pain signals can be a huge relief until you can get to the heart of the matter. But if you do this for days or weeks at a time, it is the equivalent of putting tape over the idiot light on the car's dashboard. That's right: pain medication is the same thing as ignoring the engine light, ignoring the signal completely, until the engine blows—and now we have real problems.

If we clear out the problems with the nervous system, starting with taking pressure off of the nerve roots which control all of the muscles, tissues and organs in the body, then many of the aches and pains within your body will clear up as it returns to more normal function.

Chapter 6

WHAT ARE THE SHORTCUTS TO GETTING BETTER AND ARE YOU WILLING TO PARTICIPATE?

In addition to my previously stated experience, my professional background also includes being a certified personal trainer through National Academy of Sports Medicine (NASM). These days, patients do not hire me as their personal trainer. However, my experience comes in handy when advising them on what to do. I often give them basic, core-focused tasks and home care instructions.

If you are looking to train your muscles, I would recommend seeking out a certified personal trainer who will listen to and access your needs. To recover from injuries, simple homecare is a necessity. However, simple does not necessarily mean easy. Here are the simple homecare tasks that I currently recommend to my patients:

Sleep Seven-to-Nine Hours per Night: Sleep is the most important thing I can recommend for homecare, and it is the one which is the simplest (but certainly not the easiest, as many will attest to). Sleep is so important, but so neglected, that it must be listed first. So many people are sleep deprived and are making so many bad choices due to their sleep deprivation.

Now, some people may not need as much sleep as others, but on average, seven-to-nine hours of sleep is the recommended amount of nightly sleep for adults between the ages of 18 and 64, as recorded by the National Sleep Foundation. Some individuals require as much as ten or eleven hours.

Of course, many of us aren't even getting seven hours. We have all had times in our lives where even five-to-six hours of sleep per night were simply not an option, or so we thought. Maybe we were going to school full time, raising children and working a part time job all at the same time.

But the key here is to look at your life, and break it down into smaller parts. Let's start by looking at one year. From there break it down into quarters, and from there break it down into weeks, days and hours.

I read a wonderful book entitled *The 12 Week Year*. It's a great read to help anyone get the most out of each and every day. Now, earlier in this book, I wrote about the Health Pyramid. If you recall, I placed food on the bottom, because we can live an average of 30-45 days without food. If the pyramid was made up of five levels instead of four, I would have made sleep the bottom layer. Yes, sleep is really that important.

Our optimal function will not be obtained if we do not get enough sleep. Now, if we added naps throughout the day we could probably last longer, but a person who stays awake for over 24 hours is not going to have optimal function.

So, remember, if you have spans of time where your sleep is limited, like a week or two when a big project is due, that's fine. Situations happen, and life gets busy. But in your everyday life, continuing to get so little sleep for weeks or months at a time is where we can get into trouble. Experiment with your sleep patterns and sleep times, including naps if possible, and you will feel how this has an amazing impact on your attitude and your health.

Drink Water - 1/2 your Body Weight in Ounces Daily: I know this has already been mentioned, but it needs to be mentioned again and again and again and again, because proper hydration is so neglected.

How much water does a human body need in a day? Take your body weight—let's say it's about 200 lbs.— and divide it by 2, and you get 100. That is 100 ounces of water per day for a 200-pound person. If you weigh 120 lbs., then you would drink 60 ounces of water per day.

But keep in mind, this is only a minimal starting point. If you are working outside in the heat or participating in a high amount of physical activity, then you may require even *more* water, but the above formula is a great place to start. But be careful with the sports drinks. You do not want to get dehydrated, but you also do not want to be slamming a sports drink because you pulled weeds for an hour in the back yard.

Foam Roller, for Eight-to-Twelve Minutes, About Four-to-Five Times per Week: Why? Because it is the best low-cost, accessible form of self-myofascial release or massage available today. My website, www.PetersWellness.com, has videos showing how to properly utilize the foam roller on all the different body parts. Many people know this is good for the glutes, pelvis and legs, such as the Iliotibial Band (IT Band), but they may not utilize the foam roller on their shoulders and arms where it can make a fantastic difference.

Stretching, for Eight-to-Twelve Minutes, About Four-to-Five Times per Week: In the office, we use PreCore Stretch trainers. These cost $650 - $900 each, so they are not very practical for home use. However, if you have a gym membership, many fitness centers have these machines available inside the center. If you do not belong to a fitness club, all the stretches you do on the PreCore Stretch Trainer in our office can be done at home or at the gym, even without a machine: it just takes a little ingenuity.

One form of stretching that I think is a fantastic thing to do is yoga. Take a yoga class and try it for yourself. You may be surprised at how awesome it is, not only for your muscles, but also for your mind.

Exercise Four-to-Five Times per Week: Let's start with the simple push-up. This may seem somewhat archaic to the experienced lifter or regular gymgoer. But after having been a personal trainer and having been in clinical practice as a chiropractor for over a decade, I'll tell you something: you would be amazed at how out of shape the general American population is.

Push-ups might sound easy, but new patients may find it harder than they think, and might even need to start with a modified push-up in the beginning. After that, they can work their way up to a standard push-up, over a period of six-to-eight weeks. **I expect a patient to be able to do 10-25 push-ups without difficulty after eight-to-ten weeks of beginning care**. Of course, common sense is used here, based on injury. But if your shoulder is not torn, this should be something easy to accomplish.

To paraphrase the late Jim Rohn, maybe you can only do one push-up now, but if you practice every day, doing that one plus as many as you can add, after 30 days you will be able to do more than one.

For overall cardiovascular health, the American Heart Association (AHA) recommends at least 30 minutes of moderate-intensity aerobic activity at least 5 days per week for a total of 150 minutes. At a minimum, one should get at least 25 minutes of vigorous aerobic activity at least 3 days per week, for a total of 75 minutes. Either way, you should get a combination of moderate and vigorous intensity aerobic activity. The AHA also recommends moderate to high intensity muscle strengthening activity at least two days per week for additional health benefits.

Proper Eating Daily: Now here is a topic for discussion! Let's take it back to a book I really enjoyed: *Body for Life*, by Bill Philips. This is an older book, but the information is excellent.

The first time I read this book, I saw dietary issues broken down into very simple, easy to understand and implemental terms. Eat the following way: Protein, veggies and fruit in between!

How simple is that? Again, it's just protein, veggies and fruit in between. Now, some people are fructose intolerant, and may not be able to eat the fruit. Those people will need to modify this formula. But it is no reason to throw the formula out completely. We could also make this formula much more complex, or at least go into why this simple formula works so well, but for now, let's keep it simple. Like the Nike ads say, **Just Do It.** For more detailed information on this diet, pick up *Body for Life*, or go crazy on Google and research this subject to your heart's content. But first, take action and change your life for the better with this simple change in proper eating.

Reading Time 10-30 Minutes Daily: Stimulate the mind, stimulate the body. I realize that 10-30 minutes is a large variation, but we are all at different places in our lives, and I would rather see someone read 10 minutes per day than not at all.

Let's say someone reads at a pace of one page per minute, and let's say the average book is 250 pages. This means it would take this one minute per page, 10 minutes per day person, 25 days to read this particular book. Now your reading speed may be double or triple this speed, but it gives you an idea. If it takes 25 days to read an average book, then with 365 days in a year a person could read about 14-15 books per year. I believe it was in one of Tony Robbins' books where I read, "people underestimate what they can do in one year, and overestimate what they can do in 10 years."

Let's say you are not a fan of reading a physical book. This is no longer a hindrance because we now have Kindle, Audible by Amazon and many other ways in which we can read or listen to our books. I love Audible by Amazon because I can listen to a book while I work out or drive in the car. Now, I personally prefer to read a physical book, but with the Amazon Audible app, I can also bookmark sections to go back to later, just like I do when I write, draw, scribble, and totally mark up my physical books.

I also recommend breaking up your reading into three sessions per day. A mentor of mine, Tai Lopez, recommends dividing your total reading time by three so if it is 30 minutes per day then we are looking at three ten minute sessions. He also takes it a step further, and recommends you read or listen to different types of books throughout the day. He recommends a classic book in the morning (meaning a book that is at least 50 years old). The recommended midday book would be a type of self-help book in an area that you have a peaked interest, such as the book you're reading right now. For the evening read, he recommends a biography or an autobiography.

Personally, I love this, because reading a biography or autobiography at night allows me to understand the struggles and tribulations of great men and women before me. These are people who I admired as heroes when I was growing up, and today, reading about their struggles make many of my issues seem so small in comparison; it puts things in perspective. I also love the habit of reading biographies and autobiographies at night because I find it relaxes me, and does not over-stimulate my mind before I drift off to sleep. On the other hand, reading one of my afternoon self-help books at night—such as a book by Tony Robbins or a financial book by Warren Buffett—can stimulate my mind too much, and get my brain firing on all cylinders, making it difficult to drift off to sleep.

Following the above schedule of reading has allowed me to read so many more books over the last two years, and my life has improved in so many ways. Breaking your book choices down into categories—say, health and fitness, financial education, love and relationships and personal growth—is a great way to never get bored with your reading.

When I first began reading eight minutes at a time, three times per day, I felt that it was going to be difficult to do. But I soon found that I quickly upped my reading time to 30-minute sessions, three times per day. **People are always looking for ways to improve their lives, and sometimes the simplest of things can be overlooked**. Why not learn from the mistakes and successes of others? Imagine the improvements you could make.

Try this for six months as an experiment. You will not regret it, however, remember that vision without action will lead to frustration. You must read to learn, and take time to visualize what it is that you truly desire. After that, you must, absolutely must, take massive action towards accomplishing your goals.

Give Yourself Time to Simply Think and Visualize, At Least 10-30 Minutes Daily: Taking time to be alone with your thoughts and emotions, and to connect with your inner self and subconscious mind, is highly important. Giving yourself this time to do a reality check on what you are doing and what you are working on every day is a fantastic way to improve your life and happiness.

Take the time to visualize what it is you truly want. Here is the place where we can reveal that which we truly desire within ourselves. **If this sounds challenging, then I recommend you go back to the section on Daily Reading, and read some entrepreneurial books. This will help you see that to get what you want in life, you have to know what you want from life**.

Now we all want different things, and what you want is not something for me or anyone else to judge. It is for you to know and share with others of your choosing. Maybe you want your health back, or maybe you want to make a million dollars per year or per month. Maybe you want to lose 10-50 lbs. so that you can feel alive and free again. Whatever it is, we all need to know what it is for ourselves. Otherwise, what are we doing?

If you are going on a trip, you must first have a destination. Some would say we are just going to hit the road and head west. Well, west is not as specific as it could be, but even so, it is still a destination. After we begin going to this "west," we just need to find more clarity about what we seek there. Always know, the more specific you are with what you want, the more likely you are to achieve it once you take action. Notice the key word in that last sentence: **action!**

There needs to be a time for thinking, but then we must **act** on our thoughts, visions and goals. We must take action with a phone call, a text, a journal entry of a task that will move us in the right direction, the direction towards our goals, which will help us to achieve our vision and to live our lives on purpose.

Home Traction (if needed), 15-minute Sessions Four-to-Five Times per Week, for the Rest of Your Life: The need for home traction is decided by looking at and taking careful measure of your spinal column. Using X-ray, we take measurements of your cervical, thoracic, lumbar and pelvic spine and then correlate these measurements with your subjective findings, and calculate where your traction will be the most beneficial.

Consistency in All that You Do: Have you ever started something new, like a new diet or a new relationship, but in time you realize that the newness seems to wear off—and subsequently, your enjoyment and excitement dwindle?

How do we keep this from happening in our lives? Take something simple like stretching four-to-five times per week. Now, you may be thinking that this could become monotonous, but if you keep in mind the value you get from stretching—such as less painful joints, decreased muscle pain and increased blood flow—and how these things could improve your daily life, then it becomes an activity of value. A value which can bring you more pleasure, and less pain in your life.

Remember, this does not have to be a 20-30-minute activity. Even just eight-to-twelve-12 minutes could be lifechanging if done **consistently**.

Let's look at what I have outlined below, and see how a given day may look. Let's take a busy day with a lot to do and set it into a time line. If you get into the practice of doing this, you will be amazed at how much you can get done in 24 hours. I like to chunk things down into categories, such as areas of my life, the same way I break down my goals.

Anthony Robbins does a great job of this with his training on RPM, and if you are a person who always feels that you do not have enough hours in your day, I highly recommend you look into this system of time mastery.

Another great book I read and is relevant here is *Oola* by David Braun and Troy Amdahl. They break down goal setting into the 7 F's of Oola: Fitness, Finance, Family, Field, Faith, Friends and Fun.

The following is a current day for me, and I hope it serves as a clear example of how to make this work. Of course, you can make as many changes as you want, and this is a living breathing daily plan which could be very different just six months from now, but for our purposes here, it serves to highlight what I've been discussing with you. Here is my daily schedule, with lots of detail:

4:00 am - 4:01 am: Wake up, reach over to the night stand, and grab a 20-ounce glass of water. I always set this out the night before. In the morning, I drink the entire glass.

4:01 am - 4:05 am: Walk to bathroom, go pee, and then splash water on my face to wake up a bit more.

4:05 am - 4:10 am: Put on workout clothes.

4:10 am - 4:20 am: Drive to the gym (if you don't like the gym then go to where you want to go, workout room, go outside or whatever you choose to do for your exercise). During this short drive, I give gratitude for all that is good in my life. I like to list ten things I am grateful for, and then five things that I am grateful for which have not come to be yet—but that I am actively working towards. These five things are my current goals.

4:20 am - 5:10 am: Perform workout and stretching. We can get into much more detail, but for now just know that 50 minutes is plenty of time for exercise if done properly, without wasting time between sets. More or less time is fine depending on your goals and what your workout consists of. This is also the time I will listen to a book on Audible by Amazon for about 1/2 my workout, and then I will switch over to music or financial news. Either way, I get my brain moving at the same time as my body.

5:10 am - 5:20 am: I use this time for meditation. Or, as my mentor says, "10 minutes of chess-like thinking." This time for me has become quite valuable, but that's because I've had a lot of practice. When I first started meditating, it was difficult for me to sit quietly, and just be with my thoughts. Over time, the process has become a staple in my morning routine.

5:20 am - 5:30 am: Drive home from the gym while listening to a book on audible.

5:30 am - 6:00 am: Greet, kiss, and hug everyone in my family and let them know how much I love them. Note, during the summer time, my girls are still asleep at this point, but during the school year they are up and getting ready for their day. In any case, after seeing everyone, it's off to the shower, after which I get dressed and go into the kitchen for breakfast.

6:00 am - 6:30 am: Prepare breakfast, prepare lunch and enjoy some time with my beautiful wife before the day gets away from us. During this time, I also pet and feed our kitties, as well as feeding the puppies, and letting the puppies outside for a bathroom break. Remember, you may have many things to add to your list just fit them into the time blocks where needed.

6:30 am - 6:40 am: Drive to the office. (I know some people have much longer drives than this, and some people work from home, but as I said, the schedule can be modified to fit your life.)

6:40 am - 6:50 am: Settle into my work environment.

6:50 am - 7:20 am: This is the time in which I work on whatever special project I have to work on. These projects can be anything from writing, exercise planning, extra reading, business development, trip planning or whatever I need to do for myself or my business.

7:20 am - 7:30 am: I use this time to journal my thoughts. Now for others, evening journaling might be better, but I prefer to get my thoughts out from the previous day in the morning, so I can also write out my vision for the upcoming day.

7:30 am - 8:00 am: This is another bit of time I build in for a secondary project which I am working on. (Remember, you are the biggest investment that you can make. Invest in yourself and you will be amazed at your **Return on Investment (ROI).**)

8:00 am - 7:00 pm: This is my work day. For simplicity's sake, I will not go into great detail of my work day but know that my work day is broken into many segments which allow me to work on the many different responsibilities of owning, running and growing a medical office in today's world. I also fit in my second reading time around lunch time and this can also be a great nap time if necessary, even if that naps takes place in the car or in my office chair with me feet up.

7:00 pm - 7:10 pm: I drive home with thoughts of the day. At this point in the day my energy is not the same as the early morning. This is where I begin to turn my thoughts to my family. I begin to formulate questions for my girls to see how their day was. I will check in with my wife to see how her day played out and hope that everyone is healthy and happy when I get home.

7:10 pm - 7:30 pm: Greet the kitties, the puppies, each of my girls and my beautiful wife. Sometimes this greeting is more pleasant than other times. Some days someone fell off their horse at horseback riding, got hit in the head with a ball at school, got a major bruise from the bar at gymnastics, or someone hates school because their teacher is the worst ever (our poor teachers). Whichever way this plays out, I know that sometimes life just does not go the way we may hope. This does not mean we should not plan our lives out in the greatest detail possible, we just have to accept that it doesn't always work out perfectly and that is okay.

7:30 pm - 7:45 pm: This is dinner time for me. I know dinner together is a great thing for families, but with my long work days, I have learned to spend quality time with family—and have those long, good, happy conversations—outside of the kitchen table. I want my girls to learn that conversation and togetherness does not always have to be done with food in front of us. Don't get me wrong, I love food, but our society seems so addicted to some of this stuff we call food, and so much of what we do is done surrounding food.

7:45 pm - 8:15 pm: Time for us to walk the puppies. Sometimes this is just my wife and I. At other times one of the girls will join us.

8:15 pm - 8:45 pm: This is the time for our family to hang out and get ready for bed. We can all talk more about our day, or sometimes everyone retreats to their own rooms and we all do our own thing. **I like this time because it is**

"planned to be unplanned" time. A time planned out to do whatever we all want to do or not do. Sometimes I just like to sit on the patio and listen to the waterfall in the pool and other times I may get some extra reading time, extra planning or work on a project in the garage.

8:45 pm - 9:00 pm: This is the time to say goodnight to everyone. Sometimes I feel like the Walton Family, especially when I say goodnight to the girls and then to all of our pets.

9:00 pm - 9:15 pm: This is my third time to get more reading done. I like to read an autobiography or a biography to slow my mind down as I drift off to sleep.

The above schedule gives me about 6 3/4 hours of sleep each night during the week, along with possible naps at midday, which can add another thirty minutes. This gives me 7 1/4 hours of sleep per day on average. Does it always happen this way? No, but it is my balance point. It is my point to return to in case I have to spend some time dealing with some emergency or issue which requires me to possibly be at the office later for a few nights in a row, or maybe someone is not feeling well at home and they need extra attention. Either way, this schedule gives me a reference point to return to after things get a little crazy—and they will get crazy! But thanks to this schedule, I have a baseline of balance and happiness to return to. To live an "on-purpose" life, we must live on purpose!

Chapter 7

WHAT IS WITH ALL THE EXPENSIVE TESTS?

We will only order tests that are necessary. Our office usually orders X-rays, and if further evaluation is needed, we will order a Computerized Tomography (CT Scan), MRI or MRA. Having more information is nothing but beneficial to the patient. Granted, some tests can be very intrusive when they include such procedures as radio opaque dies and barium swallows, but these tests are usually done only after some other basic tests are performed, in order to rule in or rule out the need for more advanced tests.

The hands-on exam we give in our office goes through 100 separate muscle tests to see how the nervous system is performing. Countless patients have given me feedback after going through just the initial exam process, and they always emphasize that we have been extremely thorough. Notably, that is before we have even reviewed the X-rays with them.

I would like to go into a brief overview of why some of the most common tests are done, and what we are looking for in the results of these tests.

First, let's talk about X-rays: "An X-ray is a quick, painless test that produces images of the structures inside your body - particularly your bones. X-ray beams pass through your body and they are absorbed in different amounts depending on the density of the material they pass through. Dense materials, such as bone and metal, show up as white on X-rays. The air in your lungs shows up as black. Fat and muscle appear as shades of gray. For some types of X-ray tests, a contrast medium - such as iodine or barium - is introduced into your body to provide greater detail on the images." (mayoclinic.org) This is a great description of what an X-ray is.

The information from an X-ray can allow us to see most fractures, and it gives us clear information regarding any degeneration that may have occurred up to this point.

Second, let's cover Computerized Tomography, better known as a "CT Scan" or a "Cat Scan." "A CT Scan is a series of X-ray images taken from different angles and uses computer processing to create cross-sectional images, or slices, of the bones, blood vessels and soft tissues inside your body. CT Scan images provide more detailed information than plain X-rays do." (mayoclinic.org)

Third, let's discuss Magnetic Resonance Imaging (MRI). This is a technique that uses a magnetic field and radio waves to create detailed images of the organs and tissues within your body (mayoclinic.org). "Most MRI machines are large, tube-shaped magnets. When you lie inside an MRI machine, the magnetic field temporarily realigns hydrogen atoms in your body. Radio waves cause these aligned atoms to produce very faint signals, which are used to create cross-sectional MRI images - like slices in a loaf of bread (mayoclinic.org)." Mayoclinic.org also states that, "MRI is the most frequently used imaging test of the brain and spinal cord. It's often performed to help diagnose: Aneurysms of cerebral vessels, disorders of the eye and inner ear, multiple sclerosis, spinal cord injuries, stroke, tumors and brain injury from trauma." (mayoclinic.org).

"An MRI can be done for specific organs such as the heart and blood vessels, liver and bile ducts, kidneys, spleen, pancreas, uterus, ovaries and prostate. MRI can also be very useful for bone and joint abnormalities such as torn cartilage or ligaments, disc abnormalities in the spine, bone infections and tumors of the bones and soft tissues. Because of the powerful magnets in the MRI if you have any of the following you may not be able to have an MRI at all or at least of certain parts of your body: metallic joint prostheses, artificial heart valves, an implantable defibrillator, a pacemaker, metal clips, cochlear implants, a bullet, shrapnel or any other type of metal fragment." (mayoclinic.org). MRIs are usually done after X-rays and are very useful with diagnosing shoulder injuries, or radiating spinal injuries such as sciatica or another radiculopathy.

    I have had many patients come in with shoulder pain which has been on and off for five to twenty years. Many have never had an MRI to see if they have a tear. Many of these shoulder issues can be cleared up within a few weeks but if not, a simple MRI can give us very valuable information. Many people feel MRI's are expensive, but here's a little-known tip: if you pay cash for the service at a local imaging center, they usually will give you discounted rates for cash payments, because they do not have to deal with waiting on the insurance company to pay them.

Chapter 8

WHAT IS THE STURCTURAL FOUNDATION OF THE HUMAN FRAME?

We have 26 bones in each foot; with both feet put together, that is 52 bones just in our feet. This means that 25% of the bones in our bodies are in our feet. We also have 38 muscles and tendons in our feet, along with 66 joints, and 214 ligaments. Addressing the biomechanics of my patient's feet is critical to the long-term effects of the care they receive. If you are not convinced, read on. **Leonardo Da Vinci called the foot "a masterpiece of engineering and a work of art." So, let us treat our feet as such, and they will serve us well.**

Let's break out the car analogy again. Have you ever had the experience where either your steering wheel shakes and shutters back and forth while you are driving at certain speeds? Or, similarly but different, maybe you've experienced times where the steering wheel pulls to the left or to the right and you have to fight the steering wheel to keep the car between the lines? Now with both of these cases, the cause of each issue is very different—but where they are similar is that in both cases, we are talking about a resultant problem which is felt by the driver *through* the steering wheel.

Now, we all know the steering wheel itself is not the problem. However, experience tells us that the steering wheel, where we notice the problem or symptom, is not the cause of the problem or symptom, but it is the resultant effect of an underlying true cause, such as either a wheel alignment issue or a tire balance issue.

Now let's say we bring this automobile into our friendly neighborhood mechanic. Let's say that we explain in great detail the history of the automobile, where we purchased it, how many oil changes it has had, the amazing $375 a piece tires we purchased, how we never abuse the vehicle, how we have the tires rotated every 5,000 miles and how for some reason the steering wheel is letting us know that something is wrong.

Now, imagine that he told you he was going to check the steering wheel itself and likely replace or adjust the faulty steering wheel. If a mechanic told us that, we would all get back in the vehicle and drive to the next shop. This is because we know the issues or symptoms described above are not a result of a faulty steering wheel, but rather, a deeper more foundational issue with the alignment of the wheels, or the balance of the tires or both.

Using the above analogy, you might go to a doctor for knee or hip pain which seems to have started for no reason. Perhaps it was just a gradual onset with no specific trauma to the hip or knee, but you notice that when walking for a short period, or standing in one place for more than ten minutes, that your knee(s) or hip(s) hurt as if there is something wrong within the joint. It could be a dull ache, or sharp shooting pain. We could and should look directly into the area of pain to make sure all is okay in and around the joints of the knees and hips.

But what about the foundation of these joints? What about the feet?

Never forget, our feet are our foundation. As I noted above there are 52 bones in our feet which is 25% of the bones in our bodies. Imagine if I told you I could get you a return of 25% on a financial investment? Well, when it comes to your body, you *can* get a 25% return or even greater when you get your feet properly adjusted.

As a chiropractor, if I am already going to adjust the patient, why not take the extra time to access their feet — and clear out their nervous system from the ground up? I would expect nothing less from my mechanic, or someone working in my home. If I had a crack in the wall, I would want them to make sure it is just a settlement issue, and not a crack in the foundation which would make repairing the drywall or stucco damage a waste of time until the foundational issue is addressed first.

By adjusting my patient's feet, I am giving more than what is expected and this is what makes someone stand out from the crowd of others who may be as qualified but not as thorough or caring enough to give more than what is expected.

Chapter 9

IN WHAT POSITION SHOULD I BE SLEEPING?

Let me warn you, you may not like the answer to this question: most people should sleep on their back with a pillow under their knees to help relax the muscles of the low back.

Now for some people, back-sleeping is simply impossible, for a multitude of reasons. But with that being said, let's discuss why most of us should be sleeping on our backs.

Here's the main reason why. The blood supply to the spinal cord is on the cord's anterior surface, or towards the front of our bodies. We spend a lot of time sitting in our daily lives. I remember learning in cadaver studies, older people's spinal cords have been found partially adhered to the anterior portion of the neural canal. You don't want that for yourself.

This is terrible. Can you imagine the information highway of your entire body not moving and functioning well due to adhesions to the surrounding structures? Things like this are why so many of my patients have said, "It's hell getting old." But it does not have to be that way.

By laying on our backs during sleep, we allow the spinal cord to fall away from the front of the spinal canal and we also allow increased blood flow to the cord itself. Increased blood flow means increased oxygen to the organs and tissues that the blood serves. This is a good thing, a very good thing.

Chapter 10

WHAT DO YOU THE READER WANT AND HOW CAN I HELP YOU GET WHAT YOU TRULY DESIRE??

I have used five different professional coaches over the past 13 years. After all, if even the most extraordinary athletes in the world need a coach, then why wouldn't I want to use a coach to help grow my business?

One thing I have realized during this whole process of growing my business, is that it is not the *business* which needs to grow: it is, and always will be, me who needs to grow.

If we improve upon ourselves, we will grow, and everything around us will *also* respond to this growth. This is what "coaching" actually is, in my opinion: to help someone be accountable to themselves. But to do this, a person must first have a vision of what they truly desire. If you don't know what you want, then someone else will have to decide for you.

Now for some people, they'd rather have someone else make their decisions. **Some people just want to be cared for, and not have to put in more effort than is required. But we should all want more from life than to just *survive*. We should want to *thrive*. We should want to live a life of true meaning and passion.**

So, we should all dig deep, and figure out what it is that we truly desire.

There are many books and websites which can help you finetune your focus, and create your own passionate Purpose Statement and Vision Statement. But for now, let me help you come up with a structural foundation—like the feet are to your body—which you can build upon, and make your dreams happen.

First, let's ask a question: **what is your "Why?"**

Let me explain. I was at a seminar years ago, and this question was asked—and at that moment, I finally started to understand the entire idea of philosophy. Basically, if your why is big enough, then nothing else matters.

Now, when it comes to the people coming to my office, their why might simply be that because of the pain they are in, they find themselves unable to focus on what they truly want to accomplish. Maybe pain is causing a person to have difficulty sleeping; understandably, this makes them so tired and grumpy that it effects their relationships at home and at work. Maybe someone is trying to achieve a personal record in running, gymnastics, competitive lifting or whatever it might be. But whatever your why is for getting better, make sure that you know what that why is. Build a vision around your why and create a plan to accomplish the tasks needed for you to not only reach your why—but also to create a bigger why. After that, you can help others find and achieve their why as well.

My current **Purpose (or Why) Statement** is this: I wish to share good heath, happiness and gratitude with everyone I meet. I will help reveal what people truly desire and guide them to know how being healthy, happy and grateful can lead them to achieve everything they desire.

This may look like a couple of simple sentences but they mean the world to me. Notice, I said my *current* Purpose or Why Statement. I say *current* because I feel that a person's Why Statement needs to be malleable. While my overall mission will probably remain mostly the same over time, as I read and learn more, I hope to always be able and willing to improve upon what I have written. This does not mean that it will change on a monthly (or even yearly) basis, but in two-to-three years, a word or two may change to give it even more meaning.

Looking at the Purpose Statement from above; one of my goals in designing this statement was to help eliminate **contradictions** in my life. For example, if someone comes to me because of neck or low back pain issues — and then mentions that they are eating fast food two-to-three times per week — then I feel I have a responsibility as a health care provider to help them recognize that a diet of fast food will not help them achieve the goal of less pain and inflammation in their body.

Now, I want to be careful here. I am not saying you should *never* eat fast food again. What I *am* trying to get across is that some of us need more moderation in our lives when it comes to diet. If someone is in great physical shape and they want to have something unhealthy once in a while, then they should go for it. But if you are in an inflammatory state of chronic pain, you might want to clean out the pantry, and cleanse your body of all the impurities which are causing the pain within your body.

My job, as a chiropractor, is to remove subluxations from the joints of your body. But it's important to remember that your body must heal from within. The emotional, chemical and structural stressors must all be addressed by the patient. I am not saying that without cleaning up your diet (chemical component) you will not get better, but if you *do* clean up your diet, you will feel and perform better in all areas of your life — including sleep, work and fun activities.

So, there it is. Whatever you take out of this book is up to you, but if nothing else, I do hope it has made you think about how you are living your life. Remember, you can always live your life with more passion, more happiness, more excitement and with less pain. Not because pain is bad, but because ensuring your good health and vitality are just such a better way to live.

Made in the USA
Columbia, SC
17 May 2018